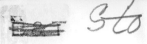

PILLS and POTIONS

**NEW DISCOVERIES ABOUT PRESCRIPTION
AND OVER-THE-COUNTER DRUGS**

PILLS and POTIONS

*James P. Kehrer, Ph.D.
and Daniel M. Kehrer*

**ARCO PUBLISHING, INC.
NEW YORK**

Our thanks to Cary Kimble, a first-rate writer and friend, whose on-target criticisms helped shape this book; to Kaye Kehrer and Debbie Kehrer for their many contributions in shepherding the manuscript, and its authors, through difficult periods; and to the American people whose ever-enlarging interest in individual health care has made the effort spent on a book such as this seem worthwhile.

Published by Arco Publishing, Inc.
215 Park Avenue South, New York, N.Y. 10003

Copyright © 1984 by James P. Kehrer, Ph. D.
and Daniel M. Kehrer

Library of Congress Cataloging in Publication Data

Kehrer, James P.
  Pills and potions.

  Includes index.
    1. Drugs—Popular works.   I. Kehrer, Daniel M.
II. Title. [DNLM: 1. Drugs, Non-prescription.
2. Prescriptions, Drug. QV 55 K26p]
RM301.15.K43   1983   615'.1   83-15826
ISBN 0-668-05717-3 (Reference Text)
ISBN 0-668-05720-3 (Paper Edition)

Printed in the United States of America

10 9 8 7 6 5 4 3 2 1

7055911

To Paul and Margaret Kehrer, the most supportive and generous parents imaginable. And to Debbie and Kaye, the most loving and understanding of authors' wives.

CONTENTS

PART 2

PREFACE

Like most Americans, you're probably not taking health care, and drugs in particular, for granted anymore. Things are changing rapidly, and the stakes are too high for you not to be informed about what is available, why it is used, what the dangers are, and what may soon replace it. If you take medicine for just about anything, you're involved. If you don't, chances are that you will at some point, and you should know what's going on.

This book puts you in touch with the latest trends, the newest discoveries in drugs. It could involve something you have in your medicine cabinet right now, or a far more exotic substance, still in the laboratory. Discover the latest in drugs to treat ulcers, pain, acne, allergies, arthritis, high blood pressure, asthma, herpes, motion sickness, infections, heart disease, cancer, hepatitis, and a spice shelf full of others. Do you take aspirin? You should know about the incredible new benefits of taking aspirin that scientists have recently uncovered. You should be alerted to new ways of taking drugs as well as about the information sheets your doctor has available and should be giving to you.

You'll find things that aren't in any other book, *because these findings are new*. Launched from our weekly syndicated newspaper column, "Consumer Drug File," this book bridges the gap between the high-tech jargon of medical science, and what you need to know about how drugs . . . *your* drugs are changing. Learn which drugs are shifting to over-the-counter status, what new contraceptives are being developed, which non-prescription products pharmacists are now recommending most, how diet drugs are proving to be a cruel myth, how generic drugs can save you money, and the latest evidence in the caffeine and cholesterol controversies. We have tried to give you the straight story, in clear terms, on these and other drug-related issues. Chapter by chapter, you'll find a briefing on each specific drug, the trends, and updates on many older drugs. Don't look for medical advice, home remedies, or an encyclopedia of pharmaceuticals here. There are plenty of those books already out there. Our aim is to bring you, the consumer, the latest information on a health care topic that greatly concerns us all. Consider this the latest report from the front.

James P. Kehrer, Ph.D.
Daniel M. Kehrer

FOREWORD

Who needs a book on the costs, risks, and benefits of medicines? We all do, and we need it badly. When it comes to medication, Americans suffer from unrealistic attitudes and a lack of useful information, a dangerous combination that can be deadly.

There can be no doubt about the importance of information concerning medicines. In the United States, the use of medicines has increased more rapidly than the use of any other health resource. Every year more than eight prescriptions are written for every man, woman, and child in this country. These prescriptions are for an ever-expanding variety of drugs as literally thousands of new medicines have been introduced in the last twenty years alone.

Non-prescription or over-the-counter (OTC) drugs are used even more intensively than prescription medicines. It has been estimated that at least forty million persons in the United States are taking an OTC drug on any given day and the actual figure may easily be two or three times this number. Several studies indicate that more than 35 percent of all Americans have used at least one OTC drug within the last 48 hours. Even the most conservative estimates suggest that there are about fifteen *billion* uses of OTC medicines in the United States each year—an average of over sixty uses per year for each and every American. With somewhere between 100,000 and 200,000 non-prescription medicines available, the complexity and pervasiveness of medicine use is difficult to overestimate.

Yet, it is our attitude toward medications, not their complexity, that is the greatest barrier to their appropriate use. Most of us have adopted two convenient illusions: We believe that prescription drugs are the physician's responsibility and that non-prescription drugs must be "safe" or they wouldn't be allowed on the market.

There is no such thing as a safe drug. All medicines have the potential to harm as well as to help and their use is based on the decision that the potential for benefit outweighs their risks and costs. That, and not simply to purchase a "safe" drug, is the decision we are making whenever we purchase an OTC medicine. Although we certainly should hold the physician responsible for using care and expertise in prescribing medicines, even with prescription drugs the individual must take ultimate responsibility for their use.

Try as we may, we cannot exclude ourselves from the decisions concerning costs, risks, and benefits of medications. Often the benefits and risks can only be evaluated in terms of our own feelings. Some of us would risk death itself to be rid of a headache, while others would prefer to let the headache go away by itself rather than to risk an upset stomach caused by pain medication. Beyond these value judgments, who but ourselves know when, where, and how medicines are used? Who else knows what foods and other medications are being taken at the same time? Who else knows whether or not there have been side effects or an allergic reaction when this drug was used previously? Who else knows what other health problems are present? Who else knows that there is a family history of problems with this type of drug? In the final analysis, only we who are using the medicine can make judgments and have access to all the information that is necessary for optimizing the use of drugs.

But we almost never have all of the information that we need to make decisions about these drugs. Before we can make a judgment as to what the potential benefits and risks mean to us, we must know what the potential benefits and risks are. Before we can avoid drug interactions with food or other drugs, we must know what these interactions are. Before we can use our knowledge of family medical problems, we must discern what parts of that knowledge are relevant to the use of drugs. We must also understand that knowledge of the risks and benefits of drugs is imperfect and that the use of drugs requires a healthy respect for the gaps in this knowledge. In short, we need information that we can use to understand the probability that a particular medication will harm or help, information that is truly useful as a basis for making a decision on the use of medicines.

Usable information on what drugs really are and what they are not is the great strength of this book. We find here page after page of information that describes costs, risks, and benefits of medications in understandable terms. The authors have walked that difficult path dictated by the facts as we know them. They have declared drugs neither all good nor all bad even though that may have been a more dramatic and salable story. But that would have been only a story, for the truth is any drug is a two-edged sword with the capacity for both benefit and injury, a weapon that we must understand better if we are to use wisely. With this book, we all take a giant step toward that understanding.

—Donald M. Vickery, M.D.
President, The Center for
Consumer Health Education

Part 1

1

FILLING THE DRUG INFORMATION GAP: ADS, TEARSHEETS, AND LABELS

Direct-to-the-Consumer Ads: A Medical First

Since the days of snake oil salesmen, medications of indescribable variety have been heavily—though not always accurately—promoted to the consuming public.

Somewhere along that trail from yesteryear came an unwritten rule in the United States that prescription drugs should only be peddled to health professionals and not directly to the people who end up using them. Drug salespeople, commonly known as "detail men," or women, display their wares to physicians and pharmacists, and the drug companies advertise only in trade journals.

That's all changing now. The first stones of this advertising barrier are being chipped loose. Brace yourself, prescription drug rebates and even coupon clipping may be on the way.

In recent years, other advertising barriers, such as those for legal services, have also fallen. Advertising prescription drugs may be next, and in keeping with the consumer movement. Accuracy of advertisements for drugs appears to be the primary concern. To be sure, physicians aren't going to like it at all, and some of their arguments will be sound. For instance, doctors are usually in a better position to know what is best for the patient and they can probably spot a bogus claim when they see it. But with some eighteen hundred prescription drugs available today, and more on the way all the time, no doctor can be familiar with every product on the market.

Although more consumer awareness of the great variety of drugs currently available will in theory aid in treatment, some doctors are already complaining that they will have to spend more time discussing the pros and cons of medications or answering questions about drug ads a patient has seen.

This could have the effect of pushing pharmacists more into the spotlight. Since drug information is their stock-in-trade, they are the ones who can help fill the knowledge gap at the consumer level. The nation's universities are now training pharmacists to assume a more active role.

Some fears about drug advertising are more disturbing. Advertising hype about cosmetics or cold remedies is one thing, but half-truths about potent prescription drugs that can raise unrealistic expectations for seriously ill people are quite another. Even if the ad is presented accurately, there might be special circumstances where the consumer lacks the medical knowledge to choose safely among competing products.

Nevertheless, several major drug firms have already broken the barrier by advertising directly to consumers, and more seem sure to follow. Consider the ads for Pneumovax (a pneumonia vaccine) that appeared in some major newspapers and national magazines, causing a stir among physicians. This ad, aimed at people over sixty-five, carried a coupon to be clipped and taken to the doctor, asking whether that doctor would inject the reader/patient with the vaccine. The problem was that studies had not conclusively shown the vaccine to be one hundred percent effective.

The Food and Drug Administration (FDA) has, at least tacitly, seemed to encourage the move toward consumer advertising. The FDA commissioner has told prescription drug companies that direct-to-the-consumer ads are actually one of the big marketing opportunities open to them in the 1980s. The FDA later backed off a bit, seeking a go-slow approach until guidelines to protect consumers could be drawn up.

The Pneumovax ad campaign was, in effect, a means of prompting patients into telling doctors what to prescribe—a novel approach indeed. Many doctors are worried that such situations will occur frequently if advertisements for prescription products become commonplace. For this reason, the FDA has regulatory powers to make sure the ads do not contain inaccurate or misleading information. If the FDA is allowed to use those powers, wholesale abuses could be prevented. In fact, the entire issue could have an added educational effect by prompting an active public debate about the usefulness of many of the medications we pump into our bodies. Companies that take an irresponsible approach could have it backfire on them with a backlash from better-informed consumers.

The approach may be through the back door, but the revolutionary move toward advertising prescription drugs to the general public could help fill a consumer information gap. Until 1982, when the Reagan administration killed the idea, the government had planned an experimental program to try to plug that hole with drug information leaflets to be enclosed in a number of widely prescribed drugs. Such leaflets, containing information about the use and side effects of a drug, would have been required with each prescription purchase. But the pharmaceutical industry fought the idea tooth and nail and the Reagan administration canceled the program.

Now the medical profession and the private-sector drug industry are trying to make up the difference by launching a variety of separate efforts to provide consumers with more easily understood information about drugs.

Some health professionals are arguing that general media advertising is not the way to pass accurate information about drugs to consumers. But in recent years, the ability to substitute low-cost generic drugs for brand-name products has given consumers and pharmacists a taste for freedom-of-choice, in a field where such freedoms did not exist in the past. Perhaps it is this ability to substitute one drug company's product for another's that has helped navigate us into the new advertising waters.

The potential for reaching consumers most interested in receiving this information has also increased with the introduction of several new health magazines and cable television channels such as Cable Health Network. Still, advertising costs money and there are fears it will only raise drug prices further.

Boots Pharmaceuticals, a British firm, may have actually started the insurrection by offering consumers rebates on a prescription arthritis medication that has been a big seller. Boots originally developed the drug ibuprofen, and sold marketing rights in the United States to The Upjohn Company of Kalamazoo, Michigan. As part of the deal, Upjohn had to go through expensive and lengthy clinical trials in order to gain approval from the Food and Drug Administration to market the drug in this country. Upjohn was to pay Boots six percent of the take.

But Upjohn neglected to secure exclusive United States rights and when the drug became a financial success, the profits lured Boots into a decision to market the drug independently in the United States, in direct competition with Upjohn.

This is where the advertising came in. Upjohn had the edge on product name recognition with Motrin, its brand name for the arthritis drug ibuprofen. In order to shoulder its way into the market, Boots had to overcome this edge. How? By advertising.

To induce consumers to switch from Motrin to Rufen (Boots's brand name), the company offered a $1.50 rebate directly to consumers on bottles of one hundred. Upjohn later said it had no plans to use similar marketing tactics, and that it considered such ads an infringement on the physician's and pharmacist's role.

Hoffmann-LaRoche, another one of the major drug companies, has also begun taking steps into the consumer advertising arena. Roche Laboratories, as the pharmaceutical division is known, distributes "how to" and "what if" booklets on different drug topics to doctors, pharmacists, and other health-care professionals for further distribution to consumers. Roche has also turned toward consumer magazines, television, and radio as new ways to go right to the public.

A series of patient information books is now being provided to physicians for distribution to their patients as a medical education service of Pfizer Pharmaceuticals. Although similar to the Roche effort, these books contain more extensive information on some specific diseases. One, for example, is titled *Learning to Live with Angina* (69 pages).

Although just beginning, such patient education efforts seem certain to expand. Instead of leading to an increasingly overmedicated society, as is possible, well-conceived drug ads might also open people's eyes to the intelligent use of items from behind the drugstore counter. Time will tell.

Patient Medication Instructions: More Dope from the Doctors

People who get a prescription from their doctor may now be leaving the office with two pieces of paper instead of one. The second item will be a Patient Medication Instruction (PMI) sheet, designed to provide more information about the specific drug being prescribed, including what it is used for, how to take it, precautions, and potential side effects.

It is a major new drug information program being implemented by the American Medical Association (AMA), the national organization of physicians in America. The AMA was one of the groups, along with the drug industry, that helped kill an earlier effort by the federal government to require warning leaflets with hundreds of prescription drugs.

This drug information program, run by the doctors themselves, is being put into effect in phases. Your physician should eventually have access to PMI sheets on about one hundred individual drugs or classes of drugs to pass along to you.

But as the AMA was emphatic in pointing out to its doctor members when first launching the program, carrying and handing out the sheets is entirely voluntary on the part of the physicians. They do not have to hand out the instruction sheets if they do not want to and recent evidence suggests that most doctors do not want to.

The PMIs are supposed to be supplemental. They are not supposed to take the place of oral instructions your doctor and pharmacist should still give you about a drug including, what it is, what it's for, how to use it, and what to watch out for.

At least for many drugs, however, you can now come away with something in writing, in case the doctor has not fully explained the medication, or if you simply forget what was said.

The AMA has also become aware that patients are now seeking more information than ever before about the drugs they take. In addition, with the increasing complexity of prescribing medications, the PMI sheets may prove helpful when distributed at the time the prescription is written, rather than after purchase of the drug, so you will have time to study it and ask questions of your pharmacist.

The format for the PMIs is a $5\frac{1}{2} \times 8\frac{1}{2}$-inch piece of paper,

PMI 002 **Thiazide Diuretics**

Patient Medication Instruction Sheet

For: _____

Drug Prescribed: _____

Directions for Use: _____

_____

Special Instructions: _____

Please Read This Information Carefully

This sheet tells you about the drug your doctor has just prescribed for you. If any of this information causes you special concern, do not decide **against** taking the medicine without first checking with your doctor. Keep this and all other medicines out of the reach of children.

Uses of This Medicine

This medicine is commonly used to treat high blood pressure. It also is used to help reduce the amount of water in the body by increasing the flow of urine. Thiazide diuretics may be prescribed for other conditions as determined by your doctor.

Before Using This Medicine

BE SURE TO TELL YOUR DOCTOR IF YOU...
• are allergic to this medicine;
• are pregnant or intend to become pregnant while using this medicine;
• are breast-feeding an infant;
• are taking any other medicine or have any other medical problems.

Proper Use of This Medicine

DOSAGE

When you begin to take this medicine, **you may notice an increase in the amount of urine** or in your frequency of urination. In order to keep the increase in urine from affecting your nighttime sleep, follow this regimen:
• If you are to take a single dose a day, take it in the morning after breakfast.
• If you are to take more than one dose a day, take the last dose no later than 6 p.m. unless otherwise directed by your doctor.

If you miss a dose of this medicine, take it as soon as possible unless it is almost time for your next dose. In this case, do not take the missed dose at all and do not double the next one. Instead, go back to your regular dosing schedule.

FOR HIGH BLOOD PRESSURE
If high blood pressure is not treated, it can cause serious problems such as heart failure, blood vessel disease, stroke, or kidney disease. Remember that this medicine will not cure your high blood pressure, but does control it. **Therefore, you must continue to take the medicine as directed—even if you feel well—if you expect to keep your blood pressure down.**

(continued on reverse side)

Precautions While Using This Medicine

This medicine may cause a loss of potassium from your body. To help prevent this, your doctor **may** want you to:
• eat or drink foods that have a high potassium content (for example, orange or other citrus fruit juices); or
• take a potassium supplement; or
• take another medicine to help prevent the loss of potassium in the first place; or
• reduce your salt intake and/or use a salt substitute.

Be sure to check with your doctor, however, before changing your diet on your own. Loss of appetite, vomiting, or diarrhea may cause a further loss of potassium and you should inform your doctor if these events occur.

Side Effects of This Medicine

SIDE EFFECTS THAT SHOULD BE REPORTED TO YOUR DOCTOR

Rare
• Severe stomach pain
• Skin rash or hives
• Irregular heartbeat
• Increased thirst
• Increased sensitivity of skin to sunlight

• Loss of appetite
• Nausea and vomiting
• Unusual tiredness or weakness
• Unexplained sore throat and fever

• Unusual bleeding or bruising
• Yellowing of eyes or skin

SIDE EFFECTS THAT MAY NOT REQUIRE MEDICAL ATTENTION

These possible side effects may go away during treatment; however, if they assist, contact your doctor.

• Diarrhea
• Dizziness or light-headedness when getting up from a lying or sitting position

• Muscle cramps or pain
• Upset stomach

The information in this PMI is selective and does not cover all possible uses, actions, precautions, side effects, or interactions of this medicine.

This PMI is produced by the AMA, which assumes sole responsibility for its content. Appreciation is expressed to the other organizations that provided assistance and information to the AMA and, in particular, the U.S. Pharmacopeia.

© 1982, American Medical Association. Portions of this text have been taken from the USP DI © 1982, USP Convention. Permission granted.

PMI 002

HDA 82-498 6/82 400M

printed on both sides. Your doctor gets them in pads of one hundred, and then simply tears one off the appropriate pad and gives it to you along with the prescription. There is also space on the PMI for the doctor to write in your name, the dosage, and other special instructions.

The AMA says it considers this three million dollar program (funded partly by the drug companies) among the most important it has ever launched. The Food and Drug Administration (FDA), which scrapped its proposed mandatory patient package insert (PPI) plans in 1982 after an uproar from the medical profession, also gave it a warm welcome.

In addition to providing basic information on drugs, the doctors group says the PMIs will help correct misconceptions about certain drugs. The AMA hopes the sheets will also promote better patient compliance with taking drugs, since a patient who understands why a drug has been prescribed is more likely to comply with the doctor's directions to take it.

Each PMI gives information on how and why the drug is used, including how to pronounce its name, things you should tell your doctor before taking it, how to use the medication correctly, precautions to take when using the drug, possible side effects (including those you should report immediately and those not requiring immediate medical attention), and information on discontinuing the medication. The AMA plans to periodically update the information sheets.

Doctors who worry about confusing or alarming patients with any mention of possible side effects were told by the AMA that particular care has been taken in the wording of PMIs to keep them simple and as short as possible, to use only commonly accepted scientific statements about drugs, and to use easily understood language. In other words, the drug data sheets are not exactly no-holds-barred statements of potential dangers in taking a drug, and may lack controversial information. They will not give you a complete list of all reported adverse reactions, since the AMA is fearful of needlessly alarming patients.

Here are twenty of the most commonly prescribed drugs, or drug classes, covered by the first batch of patient medication instructions, listed alphabetically:

- *Belladonna alkaloids and barbiturates:* Widely used for managing bowel and digestive tract problems.
- *Beta blockers:* Used in the treatment of high blood pressure, chest pain (angina), and heart-beat irregularities.
- *Cephalosporins:* Broad-spectrum antibiotics useful for certain bacterial infections.
- *Cimetidine:* Inhibits the secretion of stomach acid, and widely used in treatment of peptic (duodenal) ulcers.
- *Corticosteroids (oral):* Have a wide variety of uses, including reducing inflammation, treatment of arthritis, ulcerative colitis, among others.
- *Coumarin-type anticoagulants:* Used in patients with blood-clotting disorders and sometimes following strokes and heart attacks.
- *Digitalis preparations:* Considered primary therapy for treating chronic congestive heart failure.
- *Erythromycin:* One of the safest antibiotics used in treating certain bacterial infections.
- *Furosemide:* A very potent diuretic, used to treat high blood pressure and congestive heart failure. Effective in patients with impaired kidney function.
- *Insulin:* Essential hormonal replacement for treatment of diabetes.
- *Methyldopa:* Used in the treatment of high blood pressure.
- *Nonsteroidal anti-inflammatory agents:* Used in the treatment of arthritis, to reduce fevers, and pain.
- *Oral antidiabetics:* Used to help treat certain kinds of diabetes.

- *Penicillins (oral):* The most widely used antibiotics in treatment of many common bacterial infections.
- *Phenytoin:* A first-choice drug for treating many kinds of epilepsy, used to prevent seizures.
- *Sublingual nitroglycerin:* Used under the tongue as a drug for treatment of chest pain (angina).
- *Sulfonamides:* Widely used antibacterials for treating urinary tract infections.
- *Tetracyclines:* Antibiotics used for many common bacterial infections and also some forms of acne.
- *Thiazide diuretics:* Drugs of choice of first-line therapy in high blood pressure, useful for congestive heart failure in patients with normal kidney function.

Labeling: New Pregnancy Warning a Good Idea

It was one of those curious bureaucratic ironies that seem to plague the nation's capital. On the very day that the government's program to provide consumers with more drug information on prescription drugs was officially axed, the FDA also proposed a massive new disclosure to warn pregnant and nursing women about potential dangers in over-the-counter (OTC) drugs.

After years of waffling, the FDA has finally decided to get the word out that most, if not all, drugs can be dangerous to babies, either unborn or newly born.

No specific products that the FDA says should contain a warning have been proven hazardous to humans, but the potential danger is there. Estimates of the number of nonprescription drugs range as high as three hundred thousand, and while these products contain only about seven hundred different ingredients, the possible dangers in this number of chemicals is huge.

The government has said it wants manufacturers to put warnings on each and every OTC product containing drugs absorbed by the body. The warning cautions pregnant and nursing women against using the products without first getting professional advice about the consequences of doing so.

Basically, the fetus is exposed to whatever the mother takes. Pregnant women do take drugs, despite a growing medical consensus that this is not a good thing to do. One estimate put the average number of drugs taken by pregnant women at eleven, eighty percent of which are taken without a physician's knowledge or supervision.

Even the mildest drugs taken safely by the mother can be passed along to the child where they can affect growth and development. There's evidence that the fetus is particularly vulnerable to teratogenic drugs—any drug that can cause birth defects—in the first three months of pregnancy. Also, the central nervous system is especially vulnerable to drugs during the last trimester of pregnancy when the rate of brain growth is fastest, according to the FDA.

Testing for the specific danger to humans from the many ingredients in over-the-counter (OTC) and prescription drugs has proved a difficult, and largely inconclusive task. A recent survey found that 80 percent of prescription drugs have *no* data on their safety for pregnant women, and the situation is probably much worse with nonprescription drugs. That is one reason most doctors recommend that women avoid taking *ALL* drugs during pregnancy, if possible.

The once widely used but controversial drug for morning sickness, Bendectin, is the latest product to succumb to suspicions that it can cause birth defects. Until early 1983, when the drug's manufacturer pulled it off the market, Bendectin was the *only* drug specifically approved for morning sickness in the United States, and was taken by nearly one in every four pregnant women. Too many people, however, became convinced that the drug was the cause of birth defects, and a rash of lawsuits against the manufacturer, Merrell-Dow Pharmaceuticals, resulted. Shortly after Merrell-Dow lost one of those lawsuits, the company stopped making Bendectin, even though proof that the drug is the cause of birth defects is still lacking. Animal tests have suggested a link, but Merrell-Dow and the FDA both claimed it was safe for humans. The FDA, however, was reexamining the issue. Perhaps the underlying problem is the impossibility of proving any drug harmless—there is always some uncertainty.

Fortunately, human babies seem to be more resistant to drug-induced birth defects than are animals. For example, there is evidence that aspirin is a teratogen in mice and rats, while human studies have concluded just the opposite. Still, Tylenol (acetaminophen) is probably a prudent alternative pain reliever during pregnancy.

But this can also work in reverse; some human teratogens will not produce birth defects in rats or mice. The classic and most tragic case of this was thalidomide, which some countries gave OTC status because early studies showed it to be safe and effective, producing no birth defects in animals. The truth was learned only later when deformed children were born to mothers who took the drug.

Caffeine is an example of a chemical that has been implicated in animal birth defects, but the human evidence of danger is still inconclusive. Vaginal spermatocides have also been linked to birth defects in humans.

Not all birth defects show up as obvious physical or mental abnormalities, and some children may only have diminished physical or mental abilities. There is no telling how many children are born of average intelligence who otherwise would have been geniuses.

Despite the scientific evidence pointing to the danger of taking drugs during pregnancy, medical evidence did not finally bring the FDA to require the drug warning. Political and legal maneuvering was responsible. In the absence of a federal warning, many states were moving to require their own version. A California law, for example, would have required a label cautioning women to seek the advice of a physician or pharmacist before using OTC products. The FDA thinks other professionals can also dispense that advice and acted to head off a chaotic conglomeration of fifty different labeling requirements.

Unfortunately, the most potent nonprescription teratogenic drug pregnant women can get their hands on will not be covered by a warning label—alcohol.

The Dangers of Drugs in Breast Milk

Along with the back-to-nature movement in this country has come a renewed awareness that breast milk is best. Scientific studies have now confirmed what should have been intuitively obvious: human milk is nutritionally better for human babies than cow's milk or synthetic formulas.

Yet among this growing cadre of nursing mothers, many are not aware that most of the drugs they take are secreted into the breast milk and will be passed along to the nursing baby.

When it comes to any drug, one must remember that a baby is not just a miniature adult. Although the mother may be taking a drug that has no adverse effects on her, she can easily pass along enough of that drug in her breast milk and cause serious harm to the baby; the reason being, that a baby's liver and kidneys—organs which are meant to neutralize and excrete most drugs—don't work at full capacity yet. A relatively small drug dose ingested by the nursing mother could accumulate to harmful levels in the infant. The problem is compounded since infants are more susceptible to the effects of many drugs, making the potential harm even more pronounced.

The danger does not come only from prescription drugs either. Nursing mothers should also avoid such nonprescription items as decongestants and common pain killers such as aspirin, a factor considered in the new warning labels the FDA has required on OTC products.

A few of the more common prescription drugs that can be most hazardous for nursing infants as they are passed along through breast milk include:

- Valium (diazepam)—Moderate doses of this drug taken by breast feeding mothers have been known to produce lethargy, weight loss, and sedation in infants.
- Sulfonamides—These antibacterial drugs used to fight urinary-tract infections have the potential for inducing jaundice in nursing infants.
- Tetracyclines—These broad-spectrum antibiotics can cause permanent staining of the teeth and delay bone growth in the baby.
- Birth control pills can produce an imbalance of sex hormones in the nursing child.

While these are only a few of many possible hazards, mothers should not be discouraged from breast feeding since it is both emotionally and nutritionally the best thing available for a newborn. However, a nursing mother must always be aware that whatever she is taking can directly affect her baby.

Pregnant women receive countless warnings about the dangers of taking drugs—including alcohol and nicotine-laden cigarettes—for the unborn child. Those dangers seem more obvious for the child in the womb, and after the birth there is a tendency to feel safe about taking medication since the infant is presumably on its own.

The safest rule is: Nursing mothers should avoid drugs altogether and, if medication does become necessary, bottle-feed the baby while taking medication.

2

THE MOVE TO
SELF-MEDICATION

The Switch from Prescription to Over-the-Counter Drugs

There are two kinds of drugs. Those you can buy yourself without a prescription (OTC drugs), and those you must have a prescription from a doctor to get ($\mathbb{R}$ drugs). For the latter, you probably waited a week for an appointment, spent thirty minutes in the doctor's office, and paid him or her $25, $35, $45, or more for services rendered, often including the writing of that prescription.

We are a nation that takes lots of drugs. Doctors write many prescriptions and patients expect them to. It has become ingrained in the consumer's medical care psyche that only prescription drugs are the real thing. OTC products are often considered weaklings with big advertising budgets, put out there just to placate us and take our money.

And take our money they do. Sales of OTC drugs have topped six billion dollars per year, and have been rising twelve percent yearly, with even bigger increases expected. But what if many of the prescription drugs that have routinely proven themselves over the years were to be declared no longer the exclusive ground of the prescription writers? What if some of the best, safest, and easiest to use drugs were moved from the backroom to the supermarket or drugstore shelf?

That's exactly what is being done. Some call it a revolution toward self-medication. Many more drugs appear on the way toward the same fate. They include drugs to treat acne, coughs and colds, asthma, dermatitis, hemorrhoids, ulcers, pain, diarrhea, fungal infections, herpes, itching, insomnia, warts, and dozens more.

The era of self-medication is taking over, sparked by an increasingly health-conscious nation of consumers. Gone are the days when most people blindly march into the doctor's office ignorant of what may be wrong or how it might be self-treated, expecting an automatic prescription to cure the problem.

Attitudes are rapidly changing, from passive to active, when the issue is personal health care. One reason is that public confidence in doctors, hospitals, and virtually the entire professional health-care system has slumped. With health-care costs soaring through the roof and beyond, people are demanding ways to participate in the decisions, and to help solve medical problems on their own whenever possible.

There are many pitfalls to this trend, but drug manufacturers seem quite willing to oblige, and the FDA is also helping things along by continuing to approve the switch of many formerly prescription-only drugs to over-the-counter status.

Once called a "quiet revolution" by those fanning the flames, it may now be turning into a noisier affair. The key to keeping it within reasonable bounds is to make certain people are fully informed about the utter seriousness of taking all kinds of drugs, be they OTC medications or prescription items. There's some fear that the self-medication route will be taken too far.

Nevertheless, there's ample evidence that people are coming to like the idea of taking more personal responsibility for health care. The formula for success, according to James D. Cope, president of The Proprietary Association, a trade group of OTC drug manufacturers, is the following:

- Good products that work and that gain consumer confidence
- Complete labeling with all the information a consumer needs to use the product successfully without professional supervision or intervention
- Truthful advertising
- Ready availability of the products in a variety of stores

PANEL SUGGESTS SWITCH CANDIDATES

Shifting consumer attitudes toward drugs, and health care in general, has amazed many of the manufacturers. Some doctors even agree that there has been enough progress in the treatment of certain common medical complaints that doctors do not really need to get involved much of the time.

The trend toward taking a closer look at OTC drugs, throwing out the bad ones and looking for ways to make better use of the good ones, began back in 1972. That's when the government set up groups of experts to review the safety, effectiveness, and labeling of each one of the thousands of OTC drug products. They were also invited to suggest which prescription drugs they thought might be OTC candidates, so they did just that, citing some thirty-eight possibilities.

Since then, many others have come under discussion, and the FDA has lifted prescription-only restrictions on at least thirty. In most cases, the companies that make the products will be pushing for the switch to take place. But the FDA has surprised people and acted on its own on occasion as with its suggestion that metaproterenol, an asthma drug, undergo the switch. That action backfired on the FDA when asthma experts objected, claiming that metaproterenol could be dangerous if used improperly. After a very short run as an OTC product, metaproterenol—sold under the brand names Alupent and Metaprel—went back to being a prescription drug.

Prescription drugs often undergo improvements, making them

safer and/or more effective. At some point, a few of them may be safe enough to be considered for over-the-counter sales. Crucial to the switch would be the consumer's ability to self-diagnose the problem in order to know what to buy. The product label must then provide further information on how to use it. According to a Commerce Department projection, American consumers will quadruple the amount of money they spend on self-diagnostic kits between 1982 and 1985.

DANGERS ABOUND

Of course there are dangers in all of this. Safe and effective use of more powerful OTC products would depend in part on the ability and willingness of the drug companies to be upfront with their advertising, as well as providing accurate information on the label or in the package. If the past is any indication, many sellers of OTC products have a long way to go to prove themselves up to the task. Much OTC product advertising is still misleading, even if it's not exactly inaccurate.

Many doctors, of course, are loath to support a trend that would result in bypassing them with fewer trips to the office, even though it is clear that many visits to the doctor are unnecessary. Dermatologists, for example, were opposed to letting hydrocortisone—their biggest tool—go from prescription to OTC status.

The FDA, however, is determined to go ahead. The agency is now exploring the possibility of switching numerous drugs to the OTC category. Many of these are used for the treatment of chronic conditions, and there seems to be little need for the intervention of a doctor every time a new supply of the drug is needed.

If the increase in the number of drugs available without a prescription continues as expected, consumers will find their pharmacists taking on a bigger role. According to Dr. James Doluisio, past chairman of the American Pharmaceutical Association, and Dean of the University of Texas College of Pharmacy, "The trend toward self-medication places an increased professional responsibility on pharmacists, one which requires pharmacists to analyze each patient's condition and decide whether it is better to refer him or her to a physician or recommend a nonprescription drug."

Some examples of the sorts of drugs being considered for the switch to nonprescription status are: muscle relaxants; antibacterial agents for urinary tract infections; antiulcer drugs; and arthritis medications.

The hugely successful switch from prescription to OTC status of low-dose (0.5 percent) hydrocortisone creams, sprays, and lotions may mark just the beginning in a major change in how Americans are medicated. This switch allowed consumers to obtain directly one of the most important drugs in the entire field of dermatology. Shortly after it was given the OTC nod in December 1979, The Upjohn Company had it on the market and was advertising it on television. Hot on the trail have been some fifty-odd competitors looking for part of the $70 million that consumers are spending each year on the stuff, and saving these consumers an estimated $650 million in medical costs in the process. Consumer spending on these products is expected to soar in the next several years.

Some Drugs Which Are or May Become OTC

Ingredient	Use
aminophylline	anti-asthmatic
brompheniramine	antihistamine
chlorpheniramine	antihistamine
dephenhydramine	antihistamine, antiemetic, cough suppressant, sleep aid
haloprogin	antifungal
hydrocortisone	itching, rashes, minor cuts
metaproterenol	anti-asthmatic
miconazole	antifungal
nystatin	antifungal
pyrantel pamoate	pinworms
theophylline	anti-asthmatic

Another recent successful switch involved diphenhydramine-HCl, an antihistamine found in Benylin DM Cough Syrup (Parke-Davis), that was given the okay to go OTC in late 1981. The FDA had opposed that switch for many years. Another cough remedy, Robitussin (various compounds; Robins), although nonprescription for years, recently began selling directly to consumers rather than through doctors or pharmacists and became a highly successful OTC product with skyrocketing sales.

One side-effect of these success stories may be added pressure on the manufacturers of longtime OTC products. Facing new and tougher competition, those firms may start hitting consumers with a fresh round of "new-and-improved" reformulations and stepped-up advertising campaigns to keep their names in the public eye.

SUBTLE CHANGES

Making the switch from prescription to OTC is not always just a matter of changing the label. Sometimes subtle changes are needed to make the drug safer or more attractive to the consumer market. One such example is the anti-dandruff shampoo Selsun Blue. This highly recognized and much advertised product is the direct outgrowth of a product called Selsun that is available only by prescription for treating severe dandruff and seborrheic dermatitis of the scalp, a skin disorder.

The active ingredient in Selsun is selenium, a very toxic compound if you should happen to swallow it. Abbott Laboratories decided it wanted to get FDA approval to make Selsun a nonprescription drug. But before that could be done, the company had to lower the amount of the poisonous selenium in the product. Once that was done, however, it still was not appealing enough for the commercial market, so Abbott dumped in some blue coloring, some perfume, and some detergents, and thus a new dandruff shampoo hit the market—Selsun Blue.

Plenty of so-called new OTC products are actually not so new. The hemorrhoid preparation Tronothane, available from Abbott Laboratories for many years, is an example. It technically was a nonprescription product, but for some reason was only being promoted to doctors and pharmacists much as prescription products are.

The consumer-products division of the lab, searching for profit-making new products, rediscovered this almost forgotten preparation. They changed the name to the easier to pronounce Tronolane, put it in a flashy package, and backed it up with a big advertising budget complete with cents-off coupons. An old dust-covered product was transformed into a successful "new" product.

Many other products have followed similar routes; from Maalox (now in various new forms) for ulcers and Metamucil for constipation, to Dimetane, an allergy and decongestant product. The granddaddy of them all was acetaminophen (Tylenol). That aspirin substitute was available only by prescription from 1955 to 1960, and was not offered directly to the public until the early 1970s.

With the FDA, consumers, and manufacturers occasionally moving in different directions, it is difficult to predict just which drugs will ultimately receive approval for the switch to nonprescription status. In the near future it seems likely that several antihistamines, cough suppressants, antifungals, and a pinworm remedy will achieve OTC approval. Yet these may mark just the beginning of a true revolution in drug availability in the United States.

Mouthwash Hogwash (and Other Products That Don't Work)

For over a decade the FDA has been slowly creeping up on the makers of what are estimated to be over three hundred thousand nonprescription drug products sold in the United States. Those

OTC Products Most Recommended by Pharmacists

Category and Product	Percentage of Total Recommendations	Category and Product	Percentage of Total Recommendations
Acne:		*Arthritis:*	
1) Oxy-5	37%	1) Ascriptin	19%
2) Oxy-10	27	2) Aspirin	18
Antacids:		3) Anacin APF	16
1) Mylanta	35	*Athlete's Foot:*	
2) Maalox	16	1) Tinactin	88
3) Riopan	14	*Colds:*	
Antibiotic Skin Preparations:		1) Chlor-Trimeton D	12
1) Neosporin	46	2) Sudafed	9
2) Mycitracin	27	3) Triaminicin	9
Anti-Dandruff:		*Cold Sores:*	
1) Selsun Blue	40	1) Resolve	18
2) Zincon	18	2) Blistex	15
3) Sebulex	12	3) Herpecin-L	14
Anti-Itch/Rash:		*Cough Suppressants:*	
1) Cortaid	44	1) Robitussin	28
2) Hydrocortisone cream (0.5%), no brand	23	2) Robitussin DM	26
		3) Benylin	14

Diarrhea:
1) Kaopectate   29%
2) Donnagel   21
3) Parepectolin   20

External Analgesics:
1) Myoflex   26
2) Ben-Gay   16
3) Banalg   14

Headache:
1) Percogesic   30
2) Aspirin   21
3) Tylenol   14

Hemorrhoids:
1) Anusol   34
2) Preparation-H   23
3) Tronolane   14

Jock Itch:
1) Tinactin   65%
2) Cruex   28

Laxatives:
1) Doxidan   30
2) Metamucil   12
3) Dulcolax   11

Nasal Decongestants:
1) Afrin   51
2) Sudafed   30

Pregnancy Test Kit:
1) E.P.T.   72

Psoriasis:
1) Tegrin Lotion   35

Sore Throat Lozenge:
1) Chloraseptic   47
2) Cepastat   27

SOURCE: *American Druggist*, September 1982.

OTC products contain 700 to 800 different ingredients, many of which had never been evaluated for safety and effectiveness.

This "OTC drug review program," as it is known in Washington, where it seems to have become a permanent fixture, has already claimed many victims. More and more drugs will be added to the pharmaceutical scrap heap as the government finally brings the massive undertaking to a conclusion.

One by one the antacids (all eight thousand of them), acne products, cold remedies, dandruff relievers, pain killers, hair growers, laxatives, sleep aids, diet aids, wart removers—about seventy product categories in all—have been called on the carpet. Only about one-third of them have been able to prove themselves to be safe and effective for their intended uses. Others have been sent back for more information, while still another large group of ingredients has been quietly removed from the market. Ten antifungal agents and nine antacid ingredients were found to be unsafe or ineffective, over one hundred diet-aid ingredients were labeled ineffective, not a single digestive-aid product could pass as safe and effective, and thus it has gone. When an ingredient makes the pharmaceutical hit list, manufacturers sometimes simply replace it with something else, and consumers rarely notice. Daytime sedatives disappeared from the market when their ingredients were found to be ineffective.

One of the latest examples is oral health care products. That $1.5 billion market, including a vast line of products from mouthwash to throat lozenges, may be in for quite a shakeup. Consumers are most likely to see the changes in the ingredients that go into oral health care items, how the products are labeled, and in the advertising claims that are made for these products.

When a government panel reviewed the twenty-five active ingredients that were claimed to have a variety of uses, from pain killers to decongestants, these were some of the findings: Of the ingredients said to have antibacterial activity, none were considered safe and effective, while ten were classified as not safe, not effective, or mislabeled by the manufacturer; of the ingredients said to be pain killers, nine were considered safe and effective, while ten were classified as neither safe nor effective.

Ingredients in the products of dozens of firms were evaluated by the OTC oral health care products panel. Included were such well-known items as Sucrets, Scope, Vicks Lozenges, and Listerine, among many others.

The panel came down particularly hard on mouthwashes, saying that any claims of medical benefit and "germ killing" properties of these products are not supported by scientific evidence.

The ability of mouthwash to kill germs and prevent colds is also what sparked a lengthy battle between the Federal Trade Commission (FTC) and Warner-Lambert, the maker of Listerine. The FTC ordered the manufacturer to stop advertising that the product could kill germs that cause colds. The company's appeals were denied, and it was eventually forced to run corrective ads.

According to the report, using an antiseptic mouthwash regularly to prevent disease is "of doubtful rationality and . . . should be discouraged." The group said such advertising claims as "Kills germs by the millions on contact" and "Fast healing aid" should not be allowed.

"The absurd notion that antimicrobial agents in gargles, mouthwashes, and mouth rinses are necessary for daily cleansing of the mouth and throat is based upon tradition, promotional appeal by manufacturers, and misunderstandings concerning their effectiveness and safety," the panel said.

Antiseptic mouthwashes may even have adverse effects, yet ". . . the practice of using these agents in an attempt to relieve symptoms due to infections or to accelerate wound healing is so ingrained in the minds of both consumers and health professionals alike that attempting to discourage their use appears futile," the drug review panel said in its report.

Throat lozenges were another target. Some companies claim their effect will last two to three times longer than the lozenge itself, but the OTC panel doubts this. Panel members said it is unlikely benzocaine—a widely used local anesthetic—released from a throat lozenge could last three or four hours since a solution of the same ingredient gives only thirty minutes of relief.

Some lozenges also contain antibacterial agents that are of dubious medical value and may even harm helpful cells in the mouth and throat, according to the FDA panel report.

The ever-popular menthol ingredient did not fare well either. Its local anesthetic effect lasted only ninety seconds, and it was characterized as a "feeble" anti-microbial agent.

The panel was split on the subject of aspirin in chewing gum and other products used to soothe topical sores or inflammation. While most members said there's nothing wrong with it, a minority report claims that the topical use of aspirin in any form is "unwarranted and unjustified."

The findings of these FDA panels don't really break new scientific ground, but their reports continue to add weight to previous evidence that many OTC products do not do what their manufacturers claim.

3

DRUG DELIVERY ROUTES: GETTING IT WHERE IT'S NEEDED

New Ways of Taking Drugs

New drug discoveries often catch one's attention, but there is another revolution underway with new methods to deliver old drugs. What this vast array of pharmaceutical gadgetry offers is greatly improved accuracy in administering drugs—something that is not possible with ancient forms of tablets and capsules that are fast becoming outdated for many uses. Pills, for example, are one ancient drug dosing form that is no longer used. (What you take are technically tablets, not pills.)

One of drug therapy's big problems over the years has been the rollercoaster effect. When you first take a drug, your body is inundated with the chemical, which then quickly wears off and shoots up again when another dose is taken. The level in the body goes up and down like a rollercoaster. Many new technically advanced systems of delivering drugs are solving that problem.

Getting the drug to the specific area of the body where it is needed has been another problem that the new dosing systems are already solving. Far lower doses of a drug can be brought directly to the site where they are needed and precise levels of the drug can be maintained in the body for hours, days, weeks, and even months. For the patient, the result of this new technology is much less bother, fewer side-effects, and better results from the drugs.

Tablets, pills, needles, liquids, capsules, sprays, lotions, creams, and drops have at times all been inadequate ways of taking drugs. Stomach acid, for example, can wreak havoc with many drugs when they are taken orally. But drug manufacturers and doctors now have new drug delivery tools to work with.

Sometimes the new systems are the best or the only ways to successfully get a drug to where it is going. Other times, it has become merely a marketing ploy to get you to buy a new and improved product. Timed-release drug preparations (also called controlled or sustained-release) are one example of where the fancy new technology has been overused and overpromoted in some cases. These products, including many cold remedies, are designed to release a set amount of the drug over a long period of time, perhaps twelve hours or more. That is highly effective and useful for some drugs. For others it is not, and the beneficial chemicals will pass right through your system before ever having a chance to work. With some drugs, the effects will last a long time even without this fancy and expensive technology.

Drug-packaging engineers have come up with new ways and materials for implanting drug containers that will slowly release a steady amount of a drug. They have come up with new ways of delivering it through the skin over a long period of time, without ever breaking it, and there are a variety of drug pumps that can be swallowed or surgically implanted.

Drugs encased in microscopic capsules represent another new means of delivery. These super tiny microencapsulated drugs can then be given to a patient orally or by injection and will slowly release their contents.

One of the new delivery systems already on the market involves a drug used to treat glaucoma. A system called Ocusert uses a transparent membrane containing the drug pilocarpine, that is inserted under the eyelid and will let go of a steady stream of the drug for about a week. The older alternative is for the patient to use eye drops containing pilocarpine three to four times daily.

Contraceptives will also be using some new delivery systems. One device, implanted in the uterus, releases the contraceptive for a year, and requires a remarkably small amount of the drug compared to oral forms.

A good example of a drug that is much safer and more effective when taken by one of these new routes is scopolamine, a motion-sickness drug carrying the trade name Transderm-Scop. It is administered "transdermally," through the skin, by means of a small Band-Aid-like patch placed on the skin behind the ear. (See the chapter on motion sickness for more details on this product.)

Taking scopolamine this way, through the skin, drastically reduces the possibility of side effects that would show up if the drug were taken orally or by injection. Transderm-Scop is currently available only by prescription, but its safety and effectiveness make it a good candidate for an eventual switch to nonprescription status.

That same basic through-the-skin method is being used widely for several new nitroglycerin products to treat angina. A patch containing a twenty-four-hour supply of nitroglycerin is placed on the chest or upper arm, and will steadily release the drug. (See the chapter on heart and blood drugs for more on this product.)

An example of one old drug (around since 1965) finding new life because of a new delivery system is indomethacin (Indocin), a product of Merck Sharp & Dohme. It's an older nonsteroidal, anti-inflammatory drug that has suffered from the onslaught of newer such drugs used to treat arthritis and other pain and inflammation.

A big advantage that some of the newer drugs have over Indocin is that they need only be taken once a day. So, Merck is putting the drug into a new, sustained-release form, and giving it the new name, Indos. The new tablet, known as a gastrointestinal therapeutic system (GITS), is made of permeable plastic. Once taken, it allows in water from the body which then mixes with the drug inside the container and creates pressure that forces the drug to exit through a tiny hole in the device drilled by a laser. Proponents of the method say it can avoid the problem of peaks and valleys in the amount of drug released into the system.

All kinds of prescription drugs that cannot safely or effectively be taken in standard oral forms may also benefit from the new drug delivery technology. This could include cancer drugs, insulin, and antibiotics. Advanced tablet designs that release potassium safely have solved many of the problems with taking that substance.

Once on the market, drugs made by genetic engineering will also benefit from new delivery methods. That is because the genetically engineered products will be, for the most part, substances that break down in the stomach acid, or simply are not absorbed into the system when taken by traditional methods.

One very promising way of giving some drugs may be by using liposomes. These are essentially tiny fatty droplets that encapsulate a drug. By changing the chemistry of the fat in various ways, these droplets can be taught to seek out specific cells in the body, thus helping deliver a drug precisely where it is needed, rather than all over the body where it can cause toxic effects. Incorporating various anticancer drugs into liposomes has both increased effectiveness and decreased side effects.

Liposomes can be given by many routes. For cancer drugs, the intravenous route has been the best, while injection into muscles has shown promise as a sustained-release method for other drugs. Even the oral route has been used. With insulin, early results suggest it may someday be possible to eliminate the daily insulin injections diabetics currently must use.

Certain genetic diseases caused by the absence of specific enzymes may also benefit from liposome technology. Liposomes may make it possible to deliver the missing enzyme to the appropriate tissue in the body. For example, liposomes containing the enzyme amyloglucosidase have shown promise for the treatment of Pompe's disease, where this enzyme is deficient.

Although many early tests on liposomes look promising, the development of this drug delivery system needs more refinement. A major and as yet unsolved problem is stability. Current liposome preparations only last for one week, far less than the one to two years manufacturers would like.

Another alternative drug delivery method being pressed into greater use is through nasal sprays. With some products, a fine mist containing the drug will be easily absorbed into the body, bypassing the hazards of the stomach. Tablets can also be protected with what is called an enteric coating. This method, in use for many years, stops the tablet from dissolving in stomach acid but allows it to dissolve in the intestine, where the drug is less likely to break down and the body can begin to make use of it.

One of the most amazing advancements in taking drugs is the implantable drug pump. Several different types are being examined. One is a small device with no moving parts about the size of a kidney bean. It can be surgically placed inside a person's body and release a constant amount of a drug for two weeks or more. It's a pretty drastic procedure, but it's being tested and is showing good results when well controlled, and prolonged therapy is needed with a highly potent drug.

Mechanical drug pumps can also slowly release precisely measured amounts of a drug and get it to the place in the body where it is needed before it has a chance to be diluted or inactivated along the way. One such pump, about the size of a hockey puck, can be implanted in a person's abdomen, and has already been used in some cancer victims. Other pumps already available can be worn under the clothing and only weigh a few ounces. In some cases, these pumps allow doctors to administer a drug by way of an artery, which carries fresh blood from the heart to other parts of the body, rather than the traditional route through a vein, which is carrying blood back to the heart from the outlying regions of the body. The pumps have already been used to administer insulin to diabetics and to treat different types of cancer victims.

Capsules: Who Needs 'em Anyway?

In the fall of 1982, a shocking event involving an over-the-counter drug product rocked America. Seven people were killed when they unwittingly took Tylenol capsules that had been fiendishly filled with cyanide and placed back on the store shelf. In the wake of that poisoned Tylenol disaster, the federal government and drug manufacturers scrambled to change the way virtually all OTC products bought off the supermarket or drugstore shelf are packaged.

Makers of scores of other products had long used the packaging techniques that could easily have made OTC drugs such as Tylenol or other pain-relief capsules tamper-resistant. Why weren't the drugs already sealed in their own packages? Probably because no one thought of it.

But the overlooked question in that affair was: Why in recent years have drug companies suddenly started putting their products into capsules at all? Certainly there are some people who find capsules easier to take. But the real reason for the onslaught of capsulized drugs, when tablets were doing just fine, is more cosmetic than anything else.

Manufacturers keep changing their OTC products, such as pain killers and cold remedies, to make consumers think there is really something new, different, or better in those big, shiny, colored capsules. Usually, there is not. In fact, there has not been a new OTC pain reliever approved by the government since acetaminophen (the generic name for the drug, Tylenol, among others) was switched from prescription to nonprescription in 1960. Capsules look more impressive, cost more, and might be bigger than tablets, but the ingredients inside are the same.

If taking tablets does not bother you, there really is no reason to buy anything else. Consumers should discover that there are plenty of other ways to buy acetaminophen in generic form, for much less money. Tylenol is just the trade name for McNeil's brand of acetaminophen. You'll find the local store brand right next to the Tylenol, and probably with a similar-sounding name. The price difference can be big: $3.59 versus $1.59 for the same number of tablets at one big drugstore chain. Regular-strength Anacin III is also acetaminophen (the maximum-strength version contains caffeine), but the Anacin name jacks up the price.

Other companies, such as Sterling, the maker of Bayer aspirin, are just now coming out with coated tablets that are smoother and don't begin to dissolve immediately in your mouth. That could solve the problem some people have with taking regular tablets.

Whatever the product, it is clear that packaging changes will continue. It is a must for drug companies, as human lives and corporate fortunes are on the line. The stakes are nothing less than the confidence of the consuming public in virtually every nonprescription drug product that could possibly be tampered with.

The financial sacrifice for this confidence should not be large for consumers. New packaging methods are expected to add only a penny or two to the price of the product. You will be seeing a variety of new tamper-resistant packages since manufacturers have been given the freedom to choose among sealed bottles, plastic bubble casing for individual capsules, bands around bottle caps, vacuum seals stuck to the top of the jar, shrink-wrap plastic coverings, among others.

But just sealing the package is not enough, and consumers will also be warned on the label not to use the product if the seal has been broken or removed altogether.

The road back to sanity in the buying and selling of simple OTC products has not been a simple one.

4

THE DRUG APPROVAL MAZE: A BIRD'S-EYE VIEW

Every year, hundreds of thousands of chemicals are tested to see if they might serve some useful purpose as drugs. Out of those hoards, only a few hundred will show any promise. A scant fifteen or so out of the whole group will eventually find their way to being approved for use by the general public. The whole trip may take a decade or more. But this, too, is beginning to change.

Why do so few survive the process, and what could possibly take so long? Much of the delay involves the government agency responsible for making sure the drugs we are offered are safe and effective. That agency is the federal Food and Drug Administration (FDA), an arm of the Department of Health and Human Services.

The FDA is a classic bureaucracy, and is subject to attack from all sides. Drug manufacturers blame its overbearing regulations for what has come to be known as drug lag, meaning that most drugs these days become available in other countries long before they are sold here because of the FDA's lengthy and costly approval process.

On the other side, consumer groups, such as Ralph Nader's Health Research Group, are always after the FDA for allowing ineffective or harmful products to reach or remain on the market. They would like to see the FDA beef up its pack of watchdogs.

Since the FDA's creation in 1938 to monitor the safety of all existing and new drugs, the overall record of success is impressive, although marred by the inevitable failures. The men and women who scrutinize drugs do have a sincere desire to avoid approving something that will turn out to be harmful. That takes time, and the resulting lag has saved us from such things as the terrible birth defects associated with the drug thalidomide. Sometimes it does not work, however, and drugs are approved that later turn out to have unacceptable side-effects.

It could mean that the companies deliberately held back or misrepresented information (since the manufacturer is the one who does the testing), or that the FDA bungled it. It does happen. Most often, however, the real reason is that the trials simply did not turn up the evidence of adverse effects. Clinical trials involve relatively few subjects. People react differently to drugs and when a substance is used by the general population, side effects that went undiscovered in controlled testing may turn up. A rare, although serious side-effect may not be noticed when only a few thousand people take a drug during the last series of tests. Once millions take it, however, the problem will show up, as has happened on several occasions in recent years. With big money at stake, drug companies will also want to present their most positive information first. They may already have millions of dollars invested in development of the drug.

To help catch mistakes, the FDA runs a surveillance program on newly approved drugs to watch for unusual side effects.

Two of the most recent examples of a breakdown in the process, where the drug was approved and later pulled off the market, are benoxaprofen (Oraflex), marketed by Eli Lilly and Company as an arthritis drug; and tricrynafen (Selacryn), an antihypertensive drug marketed by SmithKline-Beckman Corporation. What should not be overlooked, however, is that both products were found to be dangerous in a short time period and were removed rather quickly before others could be hurt.

RISK/BENEFIT COMPARISONS

Every drug, no matter how seemingly harmless it is, involves risk. When you take a drug, you put a foreign substance into your body, and there are times when your body will not react favorably to it. The decision to take a drug always involves a tradeoff: Is the expected benefit greater than the potential risk?

Doctors, researchers, and other scientists often argue on the side of medical benefits, even when there are some medical risks that go along with those benefits. Politicians, consumer groups, and other segments of the population seem to want drugs as close to totally safe as possible. The issue is dropped into the laps of the regulators.

The risk/benefit ratio is involved in each drug approval decision. With some drugs it is easy. If the new product has toxic effects, and there are already other drugs on the market to treat the particular disease involved, the risks outweigh the benefits and it will not be approved. On the other hand, an anticancer drug may be extremely toxic and still be approved because the risk of not using it may be death. It is all relative.

The generic drug amiodarone, used to treat abnormal heartbeats (arrythmias), is one example. It has been available in Europe for over twenty years and would seem to be a classic case of drug lag. But other effective drugs for this are available in the United States, and besides that, amiodarone has recently been linked to a serious lung disorder called pulmonary fibrosis. In cases like this, drug lag may actually be beneficial, allowing us to look at the experience with a drug used in other countries before using it ourselves. It seems unlikely that amiodarone will be approved for use in the United States.

A MOVE TO SPEED NEW DRUG APPROVALS

The FDA has, in recent years, been taking new steps to reduce the time taken to approve a drug. The average amount of time it takes the FDA to wade through all the information supplied by a drug manufacturer is two and one-half years, and the FDA had tried to trim that to two years.

Two years is only the amount of time the FDA takes to evaluate the drug. The manufacturer will already have spent seven to ten years developing and testing it, bringing the total time from discovery to approval to a decade or longer.

It is often an inefficient system with tremendous duplication and repetition. In one move to cut back on that, the FDA has only recently said it is willing to base a drug-approval decision on evidence of safety and effectiveness gathered in foreign countries, as long as the methods used to get the information meet United States standards. In the past, all foreign studies had to be repeated in this country. That, and other procedural changes, are some of the most radical shifts in the drug-approval maze since the 1960s.

This simplifying of the maze is not taking place without opposition, however. Critics say it will mean that less safe, or unsafe drugs will have an easier time making it onto the market. In fact, that may be the unacknowledged reason that the government is also beefing up the system for drug followup—a kind of early-warning system to spot any problems.

FOLLOWING THE TRAIL

Once a compound is found to have some medical value, toxicology studies in animals are begun. The tests are done using several species of animals to give a more accurate prediction of how the drug would affect humans. If the chemical still looks safe, human testing can begin.

There is little hope of resolving some of the basic flaws in this route. For example, who knows how many so-called magic bullets have been passed over because they do not work in rats, but would have been terrific in humans!

The first tests of a drug in humans are referred to as Phase I in the FDA lingo. The basic effects of the drug are determined by testing a few volunteers who do not have the targeted disease. If nothing unexpected shows up, Phase II trials begin using patients suffering from the targeted disease. The purpose here is to find the proper dosage and check that the drug really works.

If it still looks good, Phase III trials will begin with a large number of carefully monitored patients to verify the safety and effectiveness of the drug.

All phases must be performed in sequence. They take a long time, cost a lot of money, and generate huge amounts of data. Some of the recent New Drug Applications (NDAs) submitted to the government have involved 3,000 patients and upwards of 100,000 pages of information. To cut back on that paper work mountain, the FDA is starting to request only the most important studies.

Effective notification and warning systems to detect the first sign of a problem after a drug is allowed on the market can ease much of the concern about new drugs. Before 1906, there were no controls whatsoever on drugs. That was the era of the patent medicine, when ingredients were often unknown and all kinds of wild claims were made about what the product could cure.

In 1906 a law was passed that said all drug products had to

be pure, but it still did not say anything about being safe, or doing what the manufacturer claimed. When people died from toxic drug products, safety became an issue and in the late 1930s the FDA was created to monitor the safety of existing and new drugs.

It was not until 1962 that changes in the law required that all drugs be *effective* as well as safe and set up the machinery for evaluating and approving new drugs. Since *all* drugs are toxic, striking the balance is a tough job, and one the FDA has carried out remarkably well. Drugs are chemical instruments that people use to manipulate the normal course of biological events in the body. About the only certainty is that any new drug will turn out to produce some negative effects, along with the positive ones. Intruding on Mother Nature always has its price.

5

GENERIC DRUGS: THE BIG MONEY-SAVERS ARE CATCHING ON

There is a way for you to save money, and lots of it, on many of the drugs you buy, whether they are prescription drugs or OTC medications. All you, your doctor, or your pharmacist have to do is to look for the generic equivalent.

Each year more and more consumers are putting millions of dollars back into their pockets that would have otherwise gone to the big, brand-name drug manufacturers. But it is still an easy step that too many people fail to take, usually for no good reason.

The first thing you should know is that drugs, like thousands of other consumer products, come with brand or trade names. Valium is a brand name. Tagamet is a brand name. Tylenol is a brand name. Motrin, Keflin, Librium, and Inderal are all brand names. The names of the actual chemical substances (the drug) that those brands represent are the true generic names. Valium, for example, is diazepam. Tagamet is cimetidine. Tylenol is acetaminophen. Just as Xerox, Kleenex, and Jell-O have come to stand for photocopying, facial tissue, and gelatin, in the minds of Ameri-

43

can consumers, the brand names of popular drugs have taken on similar roles.

The difference between buying one hundred tablets of Isordil (brand name for an angina drug) at about $7.80; or isosorbide dinitrate, the generic name for the same drug, at about $2.95, is 164 percent. And that is roughly the average difference between major trade name drugs and their generic counterparts, according to the American Association of Retired Persons Pharmacy Service, which keeps tabs on prices. Buying acetaminophen instead of Tylenol, even though they are the same thing, could save you money as well.

But there is a big catch to this entire generic drug movement. *A great many of today's largest selling drugs (and one hundred percent of the newest ones) are not yet available in generic form.* Why? Because the companies that discovered them still own exclusive marketing rights granted by a United States patent. Both Valium and Tagamet, for example, are not yet available generically.

When a firm comes up with a new drug, or something it believes will become a new drug, company officials file for a patent on the chemical at the U.S. Patent Office. They will also develop a catchy trade name for the commercial product.

In effect, the patent is an exclusive license to make and sell the drug for seventeen years. When the patent expires, everybody else is free to start making and selling the generic product, which would be virtually the same product as the brand-name item, except without the brand name. It will also be cheaper since the generic manufacturer does not have to repeat all the expensive but necessary safety tests. That generic product might be given another name (probably similar to the original trade name to cash in on consumer recognition), or simply be sold by the generic name of the drug.

What this all means is that the only drugs you can buy generically (and thus save money on) are the ones on which the seventeen-year patents have already run out. With more patents running out all the time, the list of drugs available this way keeps growing, and their share of the overall drug market has jumped considerably too.

Seventeen years may seem like a long time, but unless the law is changed (which is possible) the clock starts running from the time the patent is granted. It may take as many as ten years *before* consumers ever see the drug on the market. That would leave only seven years of actual exclusive marketing of the drug before it could be picked up by the generic drug manufacturers. That seven-year figure, however, is hotly disputed by the generic manufacturers who claim that the brand-name companies have more than enough time to profit from their discoveries before the patents run out.

Drug manufacturers are not generally begrudged the seventeen-year protection. In 1981, for example, the average cost of developing a completely new drug was about $77 million. Since competition is prohibited during the patent period, the company basically can charge whatever the market will bear to recover this tremendous investment and make a profit. However, there may be competition from similar, although not identical, drugs that could affect the price and three out of four new drugs never recover the initial investment. It is that fourth drug the companies are always looking for.

Anyone who thinks the price difference between generic and trade name is not that crucial should take another look. Comparison surveys of drug prices are always underway, and they continue to show that the spread between the price of the brand-name product and the price of the generic product can range from 50 percent to over 500 percent at the retail level. Manufacturers' wholesale catalogue prices to pharmacists have shown even greater price differences between the generic and the brand-name product.

It does not seem to make a great deal of sense to pay $11.10 for one hundred tablets of brand-name Persantine, a cardiac drug, when you could get the generic product, dipyridamole, for about $4.95.

Of course, if the drug you are taking is not available in generic form, you do not have much choice. There certainly is no harm in asking, and it could mean money in your pocket.

GENERIC TREND QUICKENING

Evidence is now turning up to show that plenty of consumers are asking for, and being given, generics. Doctors are doing more generic prescribing and pharmacists are telling people about generic products. In every state except Indiana, pharmacists are allowed to substitute a less expensive generic product for your prescription unless the doctor specifically prohibits the substitution. The large chain drugstores in particular have been pushing generic cost savings in recent years, more so than the smaller independent druggists. In New York, for instance, there is a chart on the wall of most drugstores, listing common medications, their generic equivalents, and the price for each.

Generic drugs are continuing to move into lists of top selling drugs each year, so that now about one in every ten of the biggest selling drugs is a generic product. If you just look at refill prescriptions, the portion now being sold as generics has soared in recent years. Comparing total sales (new and refill) of brand-name and generic drugs, the rate of increase for the generics has tripled that of the brand-name products.

These increases for generic drugs have not come about overnight. Generics have been on a steady climb since the mid 1960s, slowly claiming a larger portion of the 1.4 *billion* prescriptions that are now being filled by retail pharmacies every year.

Most of the top-selling generic drugs have turned out to be antibiotics, such as ampicillin, tetracycline, and penicillin-V-K. Part of the reason for this may be that dentists are writing more prescriptions these days, for antibiotics as well as pain killers.

With the increasing public acceptance of generics, a more favorable regulatory climate to the business in Washington D.C., and many more brand-name drugs due to come off patent, even Wall Street has been looking favorably upon generic drugs.

WHAT ABOUT QUALITY?

One of the most important questions to ask is whether or not you are getting an inferior product when you buy a generic drug. The vision of generic drug products being turned out in basement laboratories in inherently less effective form than the brand-name products they copy is simply not true. Generic drug manufacturers actually include some of the largest pharmaceutical companies in the country, such as SmithKline-Beckman Corporation and the Parke-Davis division of Warner-Lambert. Further reinforcement came in early 1983 when the U.S. Supreme Court ruled unanimously that generic drugs must have FDA approval before they can be sold to the public, even if the active ingredient already has the FDA's okay.

Having debunked the basement-factory myth, however, it should be quickly noted that all generic drugs are not created equal. *There are some bad generic products.*

There used to be even more problems until 1977 when the Food and Drug Administration moved to standardize all generic drugs, using the concept called bioequivalence. The government's requirements are supposed to assure you of getting a chemically identical drug that will also have the same therapeutic effect in the body. Different products containing the same drug are supposed to have equal bioavailability, meaning the rate at which the drug is absorbed into the body should be the same.

Of course, the drug industry has known for years that drugs that are chemically identical are not always absorbed by the body at the same rate. The difference can be caused by the different tablet binders used by the manufacturers, or by fillers added to the tablets, or simply by having different particle sizes of the drug.

FDA rules attempt to detect, and correct, any differences by requiring dissolution tests for generic tablets and capsules. They assume that if two products dissolve at the same rate that they will be absorbed into the body at the same speed as well.

Testing in animals would be the best, but such testing isn't very practical since there is a shortage of time, money, and facilities to test all the generic products. Therefore, the FDA only requires animal tests on drugs where there already is evidence of bioequivalence problems.

In reality, this means that most generic drugs get on the market without any animal bioequivalence testing. Most of the time that will not create any problems since there is a vast difference between what is a beneficial dose and what could prove toxic. A minor difference in bioequivalence between a generic and a brand-name product would not have a significant clinical effect.

Drugs with a narrow range between what is safe and what is potentially dangerous or medications that have already been shown to vary significantly are the products the FDA has targeted for testing.

In the days before the FDA regulations, many people suffered adverse reactions from generic products. The most dramatic example took place with a heart medication called digoxin. A well-known trade-name product of this drug, Lanoxin (Burroughs Wellcome Corporation), was widely prescribed and most patients were stable while taking it. When switched to generic products, some patients experienced sudden dramatic problems that were traced to a change in absorption of the digoxin from the generic product.

Since the bioequivalence rules were established, adverse effects have decreased but they have not disappeared entirely. The rules are vague, and the fact that animal testing is required only *after* problems have been documented still allows some bad generic products on the market. Grandfather clauses in the regulations that exempt products already on the market from the stiffer testing have also contributed to the problem.

Some brand-name manufacturers are even taking advantage of the differences where they exist by emphasizing in their advertising to doctors that their generic competitors do not have the same bioavailability and their medications may cause serious side effects that the brand-name product does not cause. One recent example of this is Lasix, Hoechst-Roussel's brand name for furosemide, a potent diuretic drug used for high blood pressure.

This should not scare you away from generic drugs. They are for the most part a very safe, effective, and vastly cheaper alternative to many brand-name products. If you want to save money on your drugs, the best sources of information about generic products are your pharmacist or doctor. They should know whether or not the drug you are taking has been linked to any problems. If so, that should be enough warning to avoid the substitution, in spite of the cost. They will also be able to help you select the highest quality generic product where there is more than one choice.

A STREAM OF NEW GENERICS

Since new brand-name drugs are continuously coming onto the market, it only stands to reason that there will also be a steady stream of patents expiring, resulting in more available generic products.

One of America's most popular drugs of recent years, Valium, a tranquilizer, loses its patent protection in 1985. This drug, whose generic name is diazepam, has done much for the financial picture of its manufacturer, Roche Laboratories. Manufacturers of generic brands of Valium will no doubt want to capitalize on the drug's huge popularity.

Also coming off patent in 1985 is Clinoril, the brand name for sulindac, an arthritis drug made by Merck Sharp & Dohme. The patent on Motrin (ibuprofen) ran out in 1983; and the patents on

Keflin (cephalothin), an antibiotic, and Ovral (Wyeth's brand-name norgestrel plus ethinyl estradiol), an oral contraceptive, expired in 1982.

Inderal, Ayerst Laboratories' brand name for the popular cardiac-antihypertensive drug propranolol, that has also found other uses, is losing its patent protection in 1984. Also this decade you can look for Dalmane (flurazepam); Keflex (cephalexin); Minipress (prazosin); Naprosyn (naproxen); and Tolinase (tolazamide); to become available generically, at a far lower price. This should be good news, especially for users of drugs such as Naprosyn and Clinoril, which listings of the top fifty prescription drugs show are two of the most expensive drugs to take. Another expensive prescription drug to take is Tagamet (cimetidine), but it will not be available generically until the 1990s.

PATENT EXTENSION: PUTTING GENERICS ON HOLD?

One of the hottest drug issues in Washington, D.C., has involved generic drugs and could delay the future availability of cheaper alternatives. Lawmakers have flirted with changing portions of the patent laws that have remained cast in concrete since 1861. The big guns of the pharmaceutical industry want to protect their patents longer, in compensation for the lengthy and expensive FDA testing and approval requirements. They claim that if they are to be expected to continue developing new drugs, they will have to be assured of a patent monopoly on the product for longer than the seven and one-half years they say is the effective patent life of the drug after subtracting the time it took to develop and win approval for it. The nine and one-half years lost in the slow development and approval system is time in which the companies would like to be making profits on the drug.

The generic firms disagree and contend that extending drug patent protection would only reward the companies for delays.

With a little legal maneuvering through the patent procedure, they say that drug manufacturers are already able to protect their monopolies for twenty years or longer in some cases.

The filing of patents is actually something of a chess game in the scientific business community. File too soon and you waste valuable patent protection time. Wait too long and someone else may beat you to it. Lawmakers will have to look for the right balance between the drug industry's need for incentives to continue expensive drug research and the consumer's right to health care at a reasonable cost.

TOP SELLING DRUGS

Everybody's list of top selling drugs seems to differ, depending on how the list was compiled; whether it covers both new pre-scriptions and refills; and where the figures are drawn from. The following are some of the drugs appearing on most lists of biggest sellers, although not necessarily in this order:

- Valium
- Inderal
- Lanoxin
- Dyazide
- Lasix
- Tylenol with Codeine
- Motrin
- Tagamet
- Dalmane
- Dimetapp
- Slow-K
- Aldomet
- Keflex
- Darvocet
- Actifed
- Amoxil

Some of the most common generic drugs now being prescribed include:

- Ampicillin
- Tetracycline
- Penicillin V-K
- Hydrochlorothiazide
- Amoxicillin
- Erythromycin
- Phenobarbital
- Thyroid
- Digoxin
- Nitroglycerin
- Insulin NPH
- Potassium Chloride
- Meprobamate
- Quinidine Sulfate
- Ferrous Sulfate

6

GENETIC ENGINEERING: A NEW WAY TO MAKE DRUGS

Perhaps nowhere else in the medical field has there been as much excitement recently as there has been over the new techniques called recombinant DNA technology, genetic engineering, or simply gene splicing. Through this process of programming bacteria to become tiny drug factories, many new products (and some older ones) can be made more cheaply, in larger quantities, and in purer form. In short, the potential for genetic engineering is mind boggling.

Still, the results to date—at least the variety that you can hold in your hand—have not been as impressive as many scientists believed they would be. A financial empire of genetic engineering companies, some new ones that arose almost overnight, and some started by giant corporations wanting to get in on the action, have fought their way toward commercial introduction of genetically engineered products. Some of those companies have fallen along the way.

Part of the problem, it appears, was that the bio-businessmen of the gene-snipping world overestimated the ease with which a highly advanced laboratory process could be converted to commercial ends. Producing a substance for laboratory use is one thing, but making enough of it to supply a nation is quite another.

The promise is as great as ever—we will just have to wait a little longer for the big payoff. During the mid-1980s and beyond, many improved and some new drug products made by genetic engineering will become available. The potential for many unique new products scarcely imaginable right now remains undaunted.

The idea behind genetic engineering is to snip out a piece of DNA (better known as a gene) that contains the code for a desired molecule, and sew it into a bacterium. The bacterium then uses those newly inserted genetic instructions to begin producing the desired substance (like a microscopic factory). Since the bacteria can be grown in huge tanks containing thousands of gallons of the little organisms, it becomes possible to make large amounts of a product which previously had to be painstakingly isolated from human or animal tissues. The bacteria do all the work in a fashion similar to the fermentation of alcoholic beverages.

The first human enzyme to be successfully produced using recombinant DNA technology was urokinase. This enzyme, covered further in Chapter 28, *Heart and Blood Drugs,* dissolves blood clots. Since it is a normal human enzyme, it does not cause an allergic reaction like a competing product called streptokinase. Urokinase, marketed by Abbott Laboratories as Abbokinase, is preferred, but the cost is astronomical when it is made by conventional means. Genetic engineering should eventually lower the cost of making urokinase by training the "cheap labor" bacteria to make it. (No labor unions yet in the bacterial tanks. They work twenty-four-hour shifts without complaint.)

However, Abbott has been unable to bring production of urokinase made by gene splicing up to commercial levels and the product the firm sells is still being isolated from human urine and kidneys.

One product that has made it—the first genetic engineering success to make it onto the commercial market—is human insulin. It is called Humulin and it is being made by Eli Lilly and Company, of Indianapolis, under license from Genentech, a leader among gene-splicing firms. Until the introduction of Humulin, reaching the U.S. market in 1983, insulins used here came from animals, usually cows and pigs, which are slightly different from the human variety. Human insulin, which is produced naturally in the pancreas, was not available. Its approval marked the beginning of the coming age of genetic engineering products. Initially, however, it will be more expensive than other insulins.

Human growth hormone is another product where genetic engineering holds great promise for making more available. It is currently obtained from human pituitary glands by a difficult and expensive process. The main use for the growth hormone is in treating the several thousand kids each year who suffer from dwarfism. However, when more of the growth hormone becomes available it may also find new uses in speeding the healing of burns and broken bones which otherwise do not heal well.

Genetic engineering is already making interferon more widely available as well, although for research uses only. Unlike insulin, this substance must come from humans to be effective in human patients. By training bacteria to make human interferon, scientists finally have a way of producing the large amounts needed to test interferon for medical uses. (See Chapter 31, *Interferon: Flash Gordon's Miracle Cure Comes Down to Earth.*)

The production of vaccines will also benefit from genetic engineering. The new hepatitis-B vaccine, for example, requires blood donations from people previously exposed to the virus in order to make it. If the blueprint for this product can be inserted into bacteria, a difficult and expensive step could be eliminated. With other types of vaccines, a common method is to grow the targeted disease-producing virus in eggs, which means people allergic to eggs often cannot safely use the vaccine. Here again, genetic engineering could overcome this problem by passing up the egg method and having the programmed bacteria do the job.

A similar process is being tried to produce a vaccine against both herpes simplex type I (which produces cold sores) and type II (which produces the venereal disease). Joint work of Lederle Laboratories and Molecular Genetics has already successfully induced bacteria to produce the specific herpes protein that is expected to be the basis for a vaccine. Very early work suggests that antibodies resulting from inoculations with this vaccine will kill both types of herpes viruses.

The most dramatic step of all for genetic engineering will come with the actual replacement of defective genes in humans. Disregarding the many moral issues that gene tampering has raised, this step carries the medical potential of curing many of the inherited diseases which plague mankind. Included would be such diseases as sickle-cell anemia, thalassemia, phenylketonuria (PKU), Tay Sachs disease, Lesch-Nyhan Syndrome, and Gaucher's disease.

Success in this area is probably decades away. Even when scientists find out how to insert the gene, ways will have to be found to activate it. Still more problems will then arise because the gene must also be controlled. Both too little and too much production of the missing molecule could be worse for the victim than none at all.

In the short term, genetic engineering will keep supplying us with products such as human insulin, growth hormone, and interferon. As scientists learn more, many other drugs and chemicals will be produced using the bacterial assembly lines. New ways of detecting diseases may also be found from genetic engineering as well as the means to cure them.

Genetic engineering may have raised even more questions than it has answered, but it already has vastly broadened man's understanding of how life works.

7

OLD DRUGS, NEW USES

When a drug is approved for use in this country, it is usually done so for a specific disease or medical problem. But the company that makes it often has in mind other uses of the drug—sometimes related, sometimes not—and will gather evidence to prove those other benefits. It is simple economics. The more ailments a drug can be used for, the bigger its sales are likely to be.

Although nothing officially prohibits doctors from prescribing an available drug for unapproved uses, they are usually reluctant to do so. If a drug company can convince the FDA of the additional uses for the drug, the way can be paved for doctors to begin prescribing it for those extra purposes.

The most spectacular recent example of an old drug finding new uses is propranolol. It was first approved only to treat high blood pressure but has been given the nod for use in treating angina, abnormal heartbeats, migraine headaches, a disease of the heart called hypertrophic subaortic stenosis, and a tumor called pheochromocytoma. Propranolol may also be approved for use in preventing sudden death after a heart attack.

Most of those bonus benefits were expected, based on the scientific knowledge of how the drug works. Sometimes, however, other new uses, only remotely related to the original purpose, are discovered by accident. This also happened with propranolol when researchers recently found out it could be of help to psychiatric patients. It seems that propranolol is remarkably effective in preventing the violent outbursts of rage that are characteristic of a mental disorder where the patient suddenly and without warning loses all emotional control. If the effect is verified by further studies, propranolol may benefit patients whose families are afraid to have them around because of this uncertainty.

There is also a report that propranolol can work against mild forms of anxiety. A concert pianist claimed that propranolol completely eliminated the butterflies he had always felt before a performance. The anti-anxiety effect of propranolol has apparently been known by the medical profession for several years and some physicians have secretly been taking the drug for just this purpose.

Another blood pressure drug recently reported to have some unique, totally unrelated benefits is clonidine (Catapres). One researcher claimed that it even brought life back to damaged nerves in paralyzed cats and humans. That effect is unverified, but the researcher claimed that clonidine actually allowed some of the experimentally paralyzed cats to walk again. The same dramatic results did not occur in human subjects, but they all did reportedly regain nerve sensations, including the ability to touch, to feel heat and cold, to regain bladder control and some finger movement. Researchers also discovered that clonidine can completely prevent withdrawal symptoms in narcotic addicts. How the drug does it isn't clear, but it could trigger a safe, effective, and painless way to help addicts kick their habit.

Another old drug with a new use is amantadine (Symmetrel), which was first brought to market as a flu-prevention drug. It came as a surprise when amantadine was found to benefit victims of Parkinson's disease. The drug is now available for both uses, but it is actually used more for Parkinson's disease than as an anti-viral.

Even an old standby (from 1943) found in most cough syrups, guaifenesin, is surprising people. It has been reported to help women with fertility problems to become pregnant. Since guaifenesin thins the mucus in the nasal passages, the theory is it also thins the mucus in the cervix thereby helping sperm to penetrate.

Some newer drugs are also finding additional uses. The calcium blockers, currently available to prevent angina (see Chapter 28, *Heart and Blood Drugs: A Revolution Comes of Age*) are proving to be helpful in preventing migraine headaches. This seems to be related to their ability to inhibit the constriction of blood vessels in the head, much as blocking this constriction in the heart prevents angina. One blocker, flunarizine, sold in other countries, has been reported to prevent migraine. An American doctor, in addition, claims one of his patients was helped by verapamil when all else failed.

Verapamil may also find use in treating mania. One report claimed a patient with this mental illness showed rapid and dramatic improvements when given verapamil, and rapidly deteriorated when the drug was stopped.

ONE MAN'S SIDE EFFECT, ANOTHER MAN'S TREATMENT

Looking back over the development of pharmaceuticals during the past several decades, it becomes clear that some of today's most useful products were discovered through the back door. The old saying in the drug field "One man's side effect is another man's treatment" has been borne out more than once.

An example: the thiazide diuretics are today's most widely used and safest drugs for treating high blood pressure. They were originally made as water pills that speeded up the rate at which excess fluid was removed from the body. Is there really a drug that can grow hair? In a word, Yes, and it's not new. The drug is minoxidil (Loniten), made by Upjohn. It's a highly potent, oral high blood pressure drug, and certainly wasn't meant to be a hair growth product. That showed up as a side effect, first noted nearly a decade ago. Unfortunately, when the drug is taken orally, it indiscriminately stimulates hair growth all over the body in both male and female. The problem has been in trying to control the effect. Whether a commercial product will result remains uncertain. An ointment form of the drug that is designed to localize the hair growth is being tested at several sites in the United States.

Here is another one. What do gout and penicillin have in common? The drug probenecid, another old drug that found a new use. Probenecid was first developed as a way to slow down the excretion of penicillin from the body. In the early days of penicillin, that was critical since the antibiotic was expensive and in short supply. It was also rapidly eliminated from the human body.

With the drug probenecid, doctors could give penicillin in lower doses and less often because it stayed around in the body longer.

But the use of probenecid dropped rapidly when penicillin became cheap and plentiful and it was only then that researchers discovered that probenecid would actually *increase* the rate that the body gets rid of uric acid. Since high blood levels of uric acid are what causes gout, probenecid became an effective drug to treat that disease.

When another drug, imipramine, was first being developed, scientists thought it would turn out to be an antihistamine, a sedative, or perhaps a pain killer. They turned out to be wrong on all counts, and the drug nearly ended up in the pharmaceutical scrap heap. It was only by accident that imipramine (Tofranil, Presamine, Imavate, etc.) was discovered to be a useful antidepressant drug (the first of what has turned out to be the most effective group of antidepressants in use today).

Multiple uses for a single drug are not all that unusual. It is even expected of many new products reaching the market. There is no doubt that more new uses for drugs already familiar to consumers will continue to be discovered.

8

ORPHAN DRUGS ARE
UP FOR ADOPTION

Drugs are big business, and pharmaceutical companies, like other American businesses, are out to make a profit. They are not without compassion, but there has to be a market for what they make . . . they are not in it for their health.

But what if there is not much of a market? What about the drugs to treat hundreds of rare diseases that affect only a few thousand or few hundred thousand people—not nearly enough, drug manufacturers maintain, to make developing them pay under our current system? All things considered, it might cost over seventy million dollars and take ten years to discover, develop, test, and obtain approval to bring a new drug to the market. Only about one drug in ten survives this process.

Enter the drugs orphaned by this huge fatality rate. Orphan drugs are drugs that may be useful for uncommon or common diseases, but because there is not a large enough market, no company is willing to produce and sell them. Common diseases, too, you ask? Yes, and the reason is this: Drugs made from natural substances cannot be patented. And without a patent, a company cannot own exclusive rights to the drug, and that is not profitable.

Patents also run out after a certain length of time. Curiously, if a company can figure out how to synthesize a useful natural substance, that is patentable . . . and potentially profitable.

It is no accident then, that drug manufacturers also fall victim to the herding instinct. With extremely common disorders for which millions of pills are consumed each day such as ulcers, arthritis, or anxiety, one company comes up with a better product, makes millions of dollars on it, and suddenly everybody else flocks to the market with similar drugs. It happens all the time.

Most people do not recognize the all-important step that must be made from laboratory to drugstore if a product is to be put into the hands of the user. Researchers may know of all kinds of useful substances, but before you can get them, some corporation must spend millions in research and development to get them onto the market.

Rare diseases, such as cystic fibrosis, myoclonus, sickle-cell anemia, Huntington's disease, Lou Gehrig's disease (amylotrophic lateral sclerosis), thalassemia, pyuria, pancreatic cancer, myasthenia gravis, Japanese encephalitis B, and many more do not get the attention that others do. It is a simple matter of economics. Either there are not enough people to buy the drugs or there are many people too poor to buy them, as in some diseases found only in Third World countries.

New Thrust to Spur Adoptions

With so many advances in drugs, this situation had become an embarrassment to the drug industry as well as the FDA, and the situation is starting to change. It should be noted that drug manufacturers have not completely ignored the orphans and many large firms have for years provided drugs for rare diseases at a financial loss. But these efforts are few and often involve items such as snake and spider bite potions. There are hundreds of diseases, including some four hundred which affect the nervous system alone, that could possibly benefit from orphaned products.

Private industry blames the government. The FDA's lengthy and expensive regulations for testing and approving a drug (this is the responsibility of the manufacturer) have become legend, although they have begun to loosen up somewhat. It took much public pressure and came a decade late, but the FDA finally did form a special unit to look after development of orphan drugs. They will search for potentially useful drugs that remain unavailable because of inadequate research, development, or distribution, or orphans that are not marketed in the United States. With a little arm twisting, the FDA says it will try to get a company to make and distribute the drugs they identify as potentially valuable.

Congress and the drug industry itself have also been scrambling to pick up the pieces. Drug manufacturers have formed their own group that is supposed to make recommendations about which orphans should be adopted. Just how much weight these nonbinding recommendations will have remains to be seen.

Lawmakers are also beginning to offer various economic incentives to the drug companies: liability protection for things that go wrong; tax incentives for orphan drug development; and exclusive marketing rights for natural substances. All these can do wonders for the future of drugs to treat rare diseases. Why wasn't it done earlier? Good question. Answer: Out of sight, out of mind.

A congressional study has pinpointed only thirty-four orphan drugs as being commercially available in recent years, and some of them can no longer be obtained. A good example is a drug called mapharsen. Mapharsen was once used to treat syphilis, in the days before antibiotics. No one makes it anymore, even though it's the best drug for a rare bladder disorder called pyuria.

A few other orphan drugs that have now found sponsors, according to the FDA, are as follows.

- Hematin, a product being developed by Abbott Laboratories. It is used to treat porphyria, a rare disease characterized by severe stomach pain and mental disturbances.
- L-5-hydroxytryptophan, shortened to L-5HPT, is a plant extract which seems to have the ability to correct a debilitating movement disorder called myoclonus. Since it cannot be patented, and there are only about two thousand known victims of the disease in the United States, there was no push to further develop this potentially useful drug. Bolar Pharmaceuticals has now volunteered to shepherd this drug to market, however, and victims of myoclonus may soon have a source of this useful drug.
- Carnitine is another natural product that has been ignored because it cannot be patented. It seems to help get oxygen to the heart. McGaw Laboratories is sponsoring this orphan drug.
- Ethanolamine oleate, an unpatentable drug, may be effective in the treatment of swollen blood vessels in the throat. This drug was made by Abbott until 1979 when the company stopped because it could not make any money on it. The FDA was keeping the sponsor's name confidential.
- Triethylene tetramine (trien) may be useful to treat the approximately one hundred victims of Wilson's disease who can't tolerate penicillamine, the usual treatment. Merck Sharp & Dohme has recently agreed to do the research needed to get this drug on the market.

Another orphan drug that has finally found a home is streptozocin (Zanosar Sterile Powder). This product, which has been available for testing since 1967, finally received FDA approval in 1982 following the joint work of The Upjohn Company and the National Cancer Institute. Zanosar is the single most effective drug for a rare form of pancreatic cancer that attacks 200 to 300 people per year in the United States. Recent work suggests that as many as one-third of the treated patients achieve a complete remission lasting an average of two years while another 20 percent show improvement.

These impressive benefits of Zanosar must, however, be weighed against its toxicity. Kidney damage occurs in many people and may be fatal. Thus, a careful watch on the kidney must be maintained. Other major side effects include nausea and vomiting, and liver damage.

Orphan drugs represent a difficult problem that has been sidestepped for too long. Continued public pressure can help push the FDA, Congress, and the drug industry further toward a more rational, compassionate policy. The drug orphanage is still overflowing.

9

POISON CONTROL CENTERS: HAZARD TO YOUR HEALTH?

After three decades, the effort to stop us from poisoning ourselves, and to aid poisoning victims, remains a sorely unfinished task. Underlining that failure is a new report with startling evidence that advice from local poison control centers is wrong, and even dangerous, an abhorrently large part of the time. The big losers are kids, as about half of the accidental poisonings in the United States each year affect children under five.

Ironically, the problem isn't too few poison control centers, it's too many, all of them going in different directions. As the poison control effort remains fragmented, insufficient or inaccurate information on poisonings presents a clear and current danger to us all. According to Dr. Richard Moriarty, director of the National Poison Center Network, in Pittsburgh, the greatest need in poison control today is a set of standards and procedures.

With no federal dollars for poison centers forthcoming, the improvement effort has lagged. A report in *The New England Journal of Medicine* shows us the result. Researchers, using a simulated poisoning episode, found that local poison control centers *gave out wrong information 60 percent of the time.* The consequences are tragic. By comparison, however, larger regional centers—the result of efforts to standardize and improve poison control—gave out correct treatment advice 93 percent of the time in this survey.

This grave disparity confirms the need to shift from the often understaffed, underfunded local centers to the larger regional poison centers with access to better information. The National Poison Center Network, and the American Association of Poison Control Centers are separate groups trying to consolidate the mess, and promote uniform standards among the more than 400 centers in the United States. Anybody can set up a poison control center, but that doesn't mean they'll be there with the right information when you need them. More often than not they aren't.

On the prevention side, progress has been better. Safety measures such as childproof caps on pill bottles have cut aspirin poisonings from 25 percent of all child poisonings in 1965 to less than four percent today. But many prescription drugs that should have the caps are still being dispensed without them, mostly by the smaller independent pharmacies.

A still common misconception is that vomiting should be induced in poisonings. It's true sometimes, but can also be extremely dangerous, depending on the poison. When a reliable poison center directs you to induce vomiting, the best method is a product called syrup of ipecac, available in any pharmacy without a prescription. Other methods, such as drinking salt water, are dangerous and should be avoided. Medical experts also say not to try and neutralize acid or base poisons with things such as baking soda or vinegar. New research shows that the heat from the resulting chemical reaction can cause more damage than the poison.

A list of regional poison centers is available from the National Poison Center Network, Children's Hospital, 125 DeSoto St., Pittsburgh, PA 15213. Or, ask your local center (listed in the phone book) if it has met the standards set by the American Association of Poison Control Centers.

Part 2

10

ACNE: A NEW TREATMENT FOR SEVERE FORMS

Acne: The scourge of the young. There is evidence that even King Tut, the boy-king of fourteenth century B.C. Egypt, suffered from it. It is estimated that in the United States up to 90 percent of all teenagers develop acne to some degree. It occurs a bit more often in boys than in girls.

As disconcerting and damaging to developing egos as acne may be, in most young people it will go away. But this is not the case for a small minority of teenagers who develop acne more severely than others and cannot seem to shake it.

Not surprisingly, this ubiquitous disease has spawned thousands of cures . . . most of them useless. Of the drugs and chemicals available today, the ones considered most effective are: Benzoyl peroxide, salicyclic acid, tetracycline (topical and oral), clindamycin (topical), and topical retinoic acid.

There is a new prescription product on the market that seems to be more effective against severe acne than any previous treatment. The new drug is Accutane, also known as isotretinoin, or

13-cis retinoic acid. It is marketed by Hoffmann-LaRoche Inc. This drug, which had been the subject of years of research, is taken orally and reduces the activity of oil glands in the skin, thus reducing acne.

Recent studies have confirmed a high degree of effectiveness for Accutane. Acne was completely cleared up in 84 percent of the people taking it, and the others still showed over a 90 percent improvement.

Accutane is not exactly an overnight wonder for every acne sufferer. The drug must be taken daily for four to five months to start with. Severe acne may disappear within these first few months, but it may not disappear for as long as ten months after treatment is begun. Remissions can last for years without further treatment.

Because there are some significant side effects that can go along with this drug, the Food and Drug Administration only approved it for prescription use in very severe cases of acne, referred to as cystic acne. A painful cracking of the lips was one side effect found to affect nine out of ten individuals taking the drug. Another forty percent of the people developed eye irritation, and up to twenty percent experienced elevated levels of blood cholesterol. The side effects are generally reversible once the drug is stopped, but one effect of the elevated cholesterol could be a greater risk of heart disease later in life. The manufacturer also warns that Accutane should not be used by pregnant women.

It is an effective drug, but the risks of those side effects must be carefully weighed against the benefits before it is prescribed. Accutane is also an expensive treatment. A four-month supply of the drug, the recommended regimen, goes for close to four hundred dollars at the wholesale level and would cost the patient even more at the pharmacy.

Many doctors still say retinoic acid, another prescription drug, is the most effective product available. This drug is actually derived from vitamin A (as is Accutane). It comes as a gel that is applied to the skin once or twice a day. It does not cure acne but inhibits the formation of new pimples.

A big problem is that it can be quite irritating to the skin, causing redness and even making the acne look worse for a week or two until the effects really take hold. With continued use, however, existing acne should heal and fewer new pimples will appear.

What is the cause of this emotionally trying disease? Acne is an inflammation of the oil-producing (sebaceous) glands under the skin. These glands are located at the base of hair follicles everywhere on the body, but are most active on the face, neck, and back—the most common acne sites. When, for unknown reasons, the hair follicles plug up, the glands become irritated and acne develops. The glands become more active at puberty.

The tetracyclines, a class of prescription antibiotics, are other drugs that have been used for years to treat acne. When taken orally, they inhibit the bacteria that contribute to the irritation of the glands. However, the tetracyclines affect many different kinds of bacteria and using them all the time can lead to diarrhea or more serious gastrointestinal infections. They can also permanently stain teeth if taken while the teeth are still growing.

To avoid these side effects, some of the tetracyclines are used topically. Meclocycline, sold under the brand name Meclan, is one product marketed as a cream specifically for the treatment of acne. It was approved by the FDA in 1981 and seems to be quite effective. Another effective antibiotic used topically to treat acne is clindamycin (Cleocin T). Its oral use for acne is not recommended, however, because of the potential for severe or even fatal intestinal infections.

Nonprescription acne treatments fall into three categories: Drying agents, cleansers, and medications. Drying agents and cleansers are not effective against acne. They act only on the skin surface while the problem lies deeper in the oil glands. There is even evidence that cleansers may make acne worse by irritating the skin.

Among the nonprescription medications, those containing an agent called benzoyl peroxide are considered most effective. Interestingly, this is the same stuff used in industry to bleach fabric, so you should avoid getting it on your towels or clothes.

A few years ago, oral doses of vitamin A were also promoted as an acne treatment. This turned out to be not only ineffective but dangerous as well. High doses of vitamin A can be toxic and the ill effects can aggravate acne even more.

11

ALCOHOL: THE UNRECOGNIZED DRUG

Probably the oldest drug in continuous use by man, even though we often do not think of it as a drug, is alcohol. As was pointed out recently at congressional hearings on alcohol's impact on this nation, alcoholism has emerged as the fourth most prevalent health problem today in terms of the number of people affected. An estimated thirteen million Americans are addicted to alcohol or abuse it.

With a long history of alcohol use and abuse, you might think there would be a great deal of research already done on what causes drunkenness and alcoholism and how to prevent it. There isn't. Only now are research efforts uncovering some interesting facts about this potent drug.

Although most of what we know about alcohol is negative from a medical standpoint, there always seems to be somebody looking for the silver lining, and there may even be one for alcohol. *Not* so for the alcoholic. The person who has lost control over drinking can find no benefits. For the moderate drinker, however, alcohol can provide improved digestion, relief of tension, and perhaps even a lessening of the possibility of heart attacks. Whether that constitutes sufficient reason to take a drink is doubtful. Any benefit would be modest and may be offset by an increased number of strokes, liver problems, and difficulty in driving suffered by people who drink alcohol. If alcohol consumption increases too far, liver cirrhosis and actual heart damage can occur—a condition called alcoholic cardiomyopathy.

One of the many tragic facts about the drug alcohol is that it causes birth defects as bad or far worse than those blamed on other drugs banned in this country. Children born to mothers who drank heavily during pregnancy may suffer from numerous physical and mental deficiencies called the fetal alcohol syndrome. The most obvious problems show up after heavy alcohol consumption, but there is no known safe level. The best recommendation for pregnant women is to avoid alcohol altogether.

Alcohol Myths

Researchers are finally gathering scientific evidence that points out that some of the traditional medical uses of alcohol may not be wise. Many people, including some physicians, believe that a glass of wine or beer before bed can help you sleep. However, a recent study done in Florida suggests that in elderly people with lung or heart disease a bedtime drink could cause periods during their sleep when breathing actually stops. The significance of this finding is not yet clear, but it is possible that in some people the effect could be deadly.

Another myth is that caffeine will reverse the effects of alcohol. All those cups of coffee to sober somebody up are for naught. Over the years, many sobering agents—called amethystics, because the purple gemstone the amethyst was once thought to be a remedy for intoxication—have been tested and touted. None of them work, and some are dangerous. Amphetamines, for example, can cause convulsions. But the search goes on, and new products are being introduced that may have some impact.

New Amethystics (Sober Pills)

With alcohol-related traffic deaths continuing at such an alarming rate, attention has focused on the possibility of a sobering-up pill. Since the people who get drunk in the first place do not seem to want to be sober, however, the usefulness of such an item seems to be in question.

Nevertheless, researchers have recently turned up several drugs that may someday result in such a product.

All of the potential candidates for a sobering-up drug work on the brain of the subject. One of the most interesting possibilities is a drug called naloxone. This product is already available as Narcan for the specific reversal of narcotic overdoses. Some recent evidence now points to its ability to reverse unconsciousness in a patient intoxicated by alcohol as well.

Other agents being tested for their ability to reverse the effects of alcohol are much further from use in humans. They include:

- Alphamethylparatyrosine (AMT), which seems to prevent alcohol-induced euphoria.
- Cortexolone, which may prevent tolerance to alcohol from building up in the body.
- EGTA, which may block the sedative effects of alcohol.

New OTC Sobering Products Hit the Market

While the more exotic future amethystics are undergoing experimentation, new OTC products claiming to reverse the effects of alcohol are already appearing and are receiving much publicity. They are combinations of natural substances and are said, by the manufacturers, to be non-drug products. A few medical experts have apparently been made believers, although uncertainty and skepticism still abound. Skeptics view such products as simply out to make a fast buck.

A small Los Angeles-based vitamin maker, Zoe Products, Inc., announced in 1982 that its trademark product Sober Aid had been proven to significantly reduce the physical and mental impairment caused by alcohol. Initial test results do indicate that Sober Aid may at least have somewhat greater promise than previous sobriety compounds.

The product's exact ingredients were being kept secret by Zoe, but are said to be common, natural substances. It contains no prescription ingredients. It is the unique combination that is claimed to have the sobering effects. The California Research Institute conducted drinking and driving studies with Sober Aid, and the results suggested that the product could improve a drunk's ability to function behind the wheel or at other tasks. Controlled experiments revealed an average 41 percent improvement in a variety of sobriety tests.

Since the FDA claims sobriety agents come under its tutelage, Zoe was seeking FDA clearance before marketing Sober Aid to the public.

It is important to note that although improvements were logged in tests of the sobriety aid, it is certainly not something that can completely reverse all signs of intoxication. It does not lower the amount of alcohol in the blood, and would not prevent someone from being arrested for drunk driving, nor would it protect a drinker's liver. In fact, many people fear the availability of such a product will actually encourage more drinking and driving by making people think they can drink and then safely drive if they take the sobering agent. Nobody is recommending that people drive after drinking under any circumstances. However, some of the advertising slogans, such as Sober Aid's which says "When it's one for the road make sure it's Sober Aid!" will not help get that point across.

Sober Aid comes as a powder that is mixed with water. The dose is about 10.6 grams (one-third ounce). Much more research is needed to determine the effects of lower or higher doses and to find out just what this product is doing inside the body. It seems to compete with alcohol for the attention of your brain. The manufacturer says the product takes about 30 minutes to take effect. The firm also says there are likely to be look-alike, sound-alike products coming along.

One product looking to get in on the same market is called Sober-Up Time. Here are some of the wild claims made for this product: "energizes the body . . . restores mental alertness . . . helps minimize hangovers . . . improves coordination . . . helps clarify thoughts . . . has excitatory capabilities." The ingredients listed on the box are; ascorbic acid, spirulina micro algae, papaya powder, fructose, caffeine, cayenne pepper, dicalcium phosphate, vegetable oil, magnesium stearate, and cellulose.

The chances that most sobriety products really do what is claimed appears to be minimal, even though backers will claim "scientific" studies to prove the product works. Experiments often amount to little more than anecdotal evidence, which is notoriously unreliable.

Causes of Alcoholism

Hit-or-miss research may eventually find a drug to reverse the effects of alcohol, but most people still believe the real answer will only be found when we discover why some people drink too much.

Everyone is capable of overindulging in alcohol, but only a few individuals lose control over how much they consume. Such a person is the alcoholic, and current scientific wisdom points to some type of biochemical difference in such a person's brain that may actually predispose them to alcoholism.

Just what that biochemical difference may be is not very clear yet. The discovery of a class of compounds in the brain called tetrahydroisoquinolines, or TIQs, may point the way toward a better understanding of the issue. TIQs may be formed in the brain of an alcoholic. Since the TIQs have narcotic-like qualities, this could explain why some people enjoy drinking more, and cannot control it.

Laboratory experiments have shown that TIQs can induce alcohol drinking behavior in rats, and while a similar effect in humans has not been proven, it may exist.

Predicting an Alcoholic

If alcoholics do indeed have a biochemical difference in their brains, it would be possible to predict who might possibly become an alcoholic (although not who *will* become one). Just as a test for phenylketonuria can determine whether a newborn child will be mentally retarded if not treated, a blood or urine test may someday be able to predict a genetic or metabolic leaning toward alcohol addiction.

What might the indicators be? Blood or urine chemistry changes, different brain-wave patterns, behavioral or psychological characteristics, or even food-consumption patterns could all help predict the disease. People could then be warned of the particular dangers of alcohol for them before things get out of control.

There should not be any doubt left that alcoholism is a disease. With continued research, ways to treat it effectively will be found.

12

ALLERGY ADVANCES: NOTHING TO SNEEZE AT

Allergies can be deadly, they can cause prolonged misery, or they can simply be annoying. Just ask some thirty-five million Americans who suffer allergies from a multitude of sources that are serious enough to cause them discomfort.

Medical science is not oblivious to this sizable portion of the populace, nor are drug manufacturers who have an eye on the purchasing power of so many relief-seeking consumers. As a result, drugs to tame the myriad physical discomforts of allergies are getting better, lasting longer, have fewer side effects, and will require less bother on your part in the future.

Scientists are even predicting that the 1980s will see a cure for allergies. Researchers have solved most of the mystery behind how allergies work and it is only a matter of time before some practical results will be available to allergy sufferers. Immunologists are making progress toward stopping allergic reactions at their source in the body and that is a big step beyond simply treating the symptoms.

These advances come none too soon. As our surroundings become more complex and we are exposed to ever greater numbers of chemical substances, it seems that just about everyone is finding they are allergic to something—from the mundane ragweed to such imaginative things as exercise or sex. There's even evidence that babies exposed to artificial foods early in their existence are more likely to develop allergies.

An allergic reaction is the result of an overactive or a misdirected bodily defense system. Allergies can certainly be hereditary, but that is not the whole story by any means. Symptoms range from a runny nose, to rashes, hives, asthma, breathing problems, and in the most extreme cases, such as some insect bites, even death.

The triggers for these discomforting reactions are not some strange bugs with even stranger-sounding names. They are the things you touch every day—from the dust on your television set to the nuts in your cake or a drug you are taking for something else.

The branch of medicine that fights allergies, called immunology, has had to live with a great deal of imprecision, even though the basic biochemical roadmap of an allergic reaction was discovered years ago. When the body is exposed to a foreign substance, called an antigen or allergen, a certain kind of antibody called IgE is sometimes produced. (IgE is short for immunoglobulin E). These IgE antibodies are different from other antibodies and do not seem to have much of a role, if any, in fighting disease. They are thought to be the prehistoric holdovers from earlier days in man's evolution when they were needed to battle parasites.

The IgE antibodies, looking for something to do, attach themselves to other cells in the body called mast cells. When a person who has IgEs formed during a prior exposure to a foreign substance (antigen) is again exposed to this antigen, the antibodies can cause the mast cells to eject their contents (mainly histamine) thus producing the signs of an allergic reaction.

Studies have pointed to IgE as being involved in some 95 percent of all allergy problems, and the victims will inevitably be found to have many times more IgEs in their blood than most people. Still, allergies are unpredictable, and an allergic reaction won't always occur in a person with IgE antibodies.

Antihistamines are still the most widely used allergy treatment. But all these drugs really do is block the final step in the allergic reaction, the action of histamine throughout the body. That is a great help, of course, but they fall short of addressing the real cause of the allergic person's problem. What's more, mast cells that produce the histamine can spew out other chemicals, such as leukotrienes, that are actually more powerful producers of allergic symptoms than histamine. The antihistamine drugs have no effects on these leukotrienes which may explain why they usually do not prevent all allergic symptoms.

The New Push for Better Drugs

Scientists have approached the problem of how to better treat allergies in several ways which exploit our improved understanding of what causes an allergic reaction. One idea is to develop new drugs which block the effects of all the chemicals responsible for allergic symptoms.

For years it was believed that histamine was the major cause of allergic reactions and that antihistamines could block all of these effects. But recent research points to leukotrienes as being as important, or perhaps more so, than histamine. Researchers are working on a new class of drugs called leukotriene inhibitors that may be used to treat bronchitis and asthma as well as to prevent allergic reactions.

Histamine itself is released from mast cells after the attack by IgE antibodies, while leukotrienes are formed only after a series of reactions. When stimulated by IgE, mast cells release a fat called arachidonic acid. It, in turn, is converted to powerful chemicals called prostaglandins, and to leukotrienes. Experts see no reason why drugs cannot be developed to prevent the formation of these chemicals in the body, thereby stopping the allergic reaction at an earlier stage.

Other major strides have come in the method involving a series of shots sometimes called desensitization or immunotherapy. These shots have been standard treatment since 1911, and thousands of people undergo desensitization therapy in the United States each year. At best, it provides prolonged relief from an allergy. At worst, it is a completely useless series of seventy to one hundred injections.

The theory behind this method is to gradually expose you to increasing amounts of whatever is causing the allergy—the offending allergen. This is supposed to call in the antibodies in the white hats—the IgGs which protect you from the negative effects of an allergen—by reacting with it before the bad guys, the IgEs. For some types of allergies, notably bee stings, the idea works well and can be a lifesaver. For many others it turns out to be a waste of time and money.

New desensitization techniques promise to confer protection with far fewer shots. These techniques are focusing on chemical modifications of the allergen that will increase the production of helpful IgG antibodies. Currently being tested is an allergen bound together in grapelike clumps. It appears that the same degree of protection can be achieved with ten to fifteen shots over three months that used to require one hundred shots over a three-year period.

Scientists, trying to come to the rescue, have also come up with a substance which can decrease the level of unwanted IgE antibodies in the blood. The compound, called suppressive factor of allergy (SFA), blocks the production of the IgEs. Preliminary tests suggest it can stop an allergic reaction. The fruits of this research for the everyday allergy sufferer may still be years away, but at least the outlook is promising.

Drugs That Don't Make You Drowsy

Allergy sufferers may soon have another reason to rejoice. New antihistamines that don't make you drowsy, hundreds of times more powerful than before, will soon be available. One of the drugs lasts so long you'd only need it once a day. While antihistamine drowsiness has been exploited in sleep aids, it's a big problem for allergy sufferers. The new prescription drugs may solve that.

The best appears to be astemizole, from Janssen Pharmaceutica. Studies show it to be 400 to 600 times more potent than other antihistamines. In England it's sold as Hismanal and it need only be taken once a day. Also coming is terfenadine, given the brand name Seldane by Merrell-Dow. It also avoids drowsiness, but would have to be taken several times a day. Other promising antihistamines are mequitazine from A. H. Robins, and oxatomide, from Janssen. All will probably be prescription items, but could eventually be switched to OTC status.

A word of caution: Antihistamines are not for colds and don't work against cold symptoms, even though they are widely misused by drug companies for this purpose. Manufacturers put them in cold medications to try and take advantage of a side effect, but antihistamines aren't meant for colds and may do more harm than good. For colds, a decongestant is best. Ralph Nader's Health Research Group has bluntly recommended that no antihistamine-containing product be used to treat the common cold. Only a few OTC cold remedies avoid antihistamines. These include: Sudafed (Burroughs Wellcome); Daycare (Vicks); and, Head & Chest (Norwich Eaton).

Two new cortisone compounds, bedomethasone and flunisolide, may also be available soon. They will be in a nasal spray form and are intended for people who have trouble controlling their allergies with other drugs.

A drug called cromolyn sodium, which has been used by inhalation for asthma for years (since 1968), should also become available soon as a nasal spray for hayfever sufferers. Nasal sprays to produce immunity are being tested as well and could conceivably replace the shots used for desensitization.

Once all these ideas become reality, victims of allergies need no longer suffer. In the meantime, the most effective allergy-prevention technique remains the same as always: Stay away from things that offend.

13

ANTIBIOTICS: FIGHTING
THE NEW SUPER BACTERIA

It's a vicious circle. First came the bacteria. Then man discovered antibiotics to fight bacterial infections. But the bacteria gradually became immune to man's chemical weapons. Man created new weapons. Again the disease-producing bacteria—called pathogens—responded by developing an immunity to the drugs. Then the drugs were altered again. . . .

When penicillin G was first introduced many years ago, it was able to kill most strains of the organism *Staphylococcus,* which is responsible for the common "Staph" infection. Today, as many as ninety-five percent of the Staphylococci found in hospitals are resistant to this drug.

As a result, consumers will be seeing more and more new antibiotics coming onto the market all the time. Just a few of the most recent additions include: piperacillin, mezlocillin, azlocillin, and bacampicillin, which all belong to the penicillin family. Moxalactam and cefotaxime, two other newcomers, belong to the third-generation of a potent antibiotic group, the cephalosporins.

The scorecard on antibiotics can get a bit lengthy—kind of like trying to keep track of all the players in the first pre-season game of professional football. Just bear in mind that all the antibiotics are organic chemicals that set themselves apart from one another only by various structural differences. They will all hunt down and kill the offending bacteria, but their methods of getting the job done may differ.

The two major classes of antibiotics mentioned before, the penicillins and the cephalosporins, exterminate bacteria by wiping out their cell walls. Without a cell wall, a bacterium cannot survive. Penicillins and cephalosporins only work against actively growing bacteria, and would be of little use against bacteria that are just sitting around dormant, waiting to become active again.

Other types of antibiotics, such as the tetracyclines and the aminoglycosides, kill bacteria by knocking out their ability to synthesize proteins. Without that ability, they can't grow, and when they cannot grow they will most often die. Using the football analogy again, think of the antibiotics as a large team, subdivided into smaller specialized groups, such as receivers, running backs, and linemen. Each member has a place on the team, but move him to another position, and he may no longer be effective.

Largely because of the 80 or so antibiotics now available, once fatal bacterial infections such as pneumonia, tuberculosis, scarlet fever, and cholera can be controlled. But medical science cannot rest on past laurels. The pathogens catch on too quickly.

Chemists have come through in two ways. They have modified the basic penicillin and cephalosporin molecules to make new drugs effective against the "super" bacteria; and they've come up with some entirely new classes of antibiotics. Your doctor has the option of switching to the alternate antibiotics in the face of a particularly tough organism.

But there are problems. The alternate antibiotics are often more toxic to your system and are not always completely effective against the target bacteria. Almost as soon as a new drug is introduced, highly adaptive bacteria can develop a resistance.

Another budding problem in this field is the overabundance of drugs. Many are just "me too" products that offer little or no advantage over existing antibiotics. But since they are chemically different, and can be patented, they are often marketed as major new products, which they are not. The corporate battle for pieces of the $1.6 billion antibiotic market is intense, and is another reason there are so many new antibiotics.

It is generally conceded, however, that moxalactam (Moxam) and cefotaxime (Claforan) represent a major advance in the cephalosporin class of antibiotics. Both are more effective against more types of bacteria. In particular, they are more resistant to an enzyme called beta-lactamase, which can destroy many other antibiotics of the penicillin and cephalosporin classes. Their main disadvantage is that they must be given by injection since they are degraded in the stomach.

The cephalosporins as a group account for about thirty-five percent of all antibiotics used. The onslaught of the third generation of these drugs seems certain to push that figure higher. At least three of the new cephalosporins are now available (moxalactam, cefotaxime, and cefoperazone) and as many as six more may be on the way.

Two of these newest cephalosporins which are the closest to market are cefsulodin, which is to be marketed by TAP (a joint venture of Abbott Laboratories and Takeda Pharmaceuticals, the largest Japanese drug firm) and cefonicid, to be marketed by Smith-Kline-Beckman as Monocid. Cefsulodin is unique in that it seems to work best against only *Pseudomonas,* a particularly nasty disease-causing bacteria that's hard to treat with other antibiotics. Cefonicid's big plus is that it lasts much longer than other antibiotics of this class and may find use in the doctor's office rather than just in hospitals.

As the number of new cephalosporins available increases, concern is growing over how to decide which of the new drugs is best. The differences appear minimal, and which ones will come out on top is yet to be decided.

One variable of concern to consumers is the price of these third-generation cephalosporins. The new drugs cost more than twice as much as the old ones. But for some infections, the old drug will be just as effective, if not better, than the new entry. New, in the field of antibiotics, does not always imply better.

The four new products in the penicillin family all come with few toxic side effects, although allergic reactions can still occur and should be watched for. Both piperacillin (Pipracil) and bacampicillin (Spectrobid) are derivatives of ampicillin, which is itself a derivative of penicillin. Mezlocillin (Mezlin) and azlocillin (Azlin) are structurally different but still relatives of penicillin.

Mezlin, Azlin, and Pipracil kill more kinds of bacteria than ampicillin, particularly the dangerous *Pseudomonas* species. But each of these antibiotics must be given by injection. Spectrobid, on the other hand, may be used orally. Once inside the body it is metabolized to ampicillin which then serves as the active antibiotic. That means its only real advantage over regular ampicillin is its better absorption and the ability to take it less often. You may not even want to bother learning the names of these drugs as replacements may be soon ready for the market.

A Forgotten Class of Antibiotics

These days, hardly a month goes by without news of some new antibiotic. But while there have been plenty of improved penicillin and cephalosporin derivatives, advances in other classes of antibiotics have been few and far between. This is especially true of the aminoglycoside class of antibiotics, which counts streptomycin as a member. Gentamicin and tobramycin are the most widely used antibiotics in this class today.

The big problem with aminoglycoside drugs is their tendency

to cause hearing loss and balance problems, not to mention kidney damage in up to two percent of the people taking them.

The new development here has occurred at Schering Laboratories, which has received approval for a new aminoglycoside called netilmicin, and given the trade name Netromycin. Both human and animal studies have shown very little hearing loss or disturbances in balance. Kidney damage is also much less of a problem, but liver damage, an effect not seen with other antibiotics of this type, may occur.

Until now, the severe, and often irreversible side effects of antibiotics in the aminoglycoside class argued against their use. But they can be life savers in some situations, and taken together with penicillins or cephalosporins they can be even more effective in curing previously fatal infections. Don't forget that after 1940, it was streptomycin that almost singlehandedly chopped tuberculosis from the list of the top ten killers.

The addition of netilmicin has made using the aminoglycosides much safer, and it may eventually become the drug-of-choice for doctors needing an antibiotic in this class. In the meantime, other drugs of this class are being studied and may offer further improvements. Furthest along are sagamicin, which has been tested in humans in Japan, and o-demethyl fortimicin from Abbott Laboratories which, like netilmicin is less toxic than other drugs in this class.

The sad part of this is that we are sorely going to need these new antibiotics in a steady stream. The way antibiotics are indiscriminately overused is feeding the fire of bacterial mutations. The more antibiotics are used (unwisely in many cases), the more chances the bacteria have to improve their defenses—and that is exactly what they've been doing. The practice of feeding massive amounts of antibiotics to livestock to increase their ability to gain weight quickly has also contributed greatly to the creation of the new super bacteria that can thumb their noses at the once-effective antibiotics.

New Bacterial Infections: An Underrated Medical Problem

People are dying in the United States because their bacterial infections will no longer succumb to the standard antibiotics. Bacterial infections are one of the leading causes of death in the United States, as the rare infections become the common ones.

Yet, the general public, conditioned by years of medical miracles and the eradication of some diseases from the face of the earth, often seems to downplay the potential dangers of common infections. There are hundreds of different kinds, posing a serious health threat that can be too easily swept aside in the face of the bigger medical problems, such as cancer and heart disease.

For antibiotic triumphs to continue, drug manufacturers will have to find out still more about how the tricky bacteria do it. They all seem to have a different method. The amazing bacterial "jumping gene," for example, can apparently communicate the secret code of antibiotic resistance from one type of bacteria to another.

Penicillins and cephalosporins (together known as beta-lactam antibiotics) are two of the safest and most widely prescribed groups of antibiotics. A big problem with the beta-lactam-type antibiotics, however, is their vulnerability to the beta-lactamase enzyme. This enzyme, produced by some of those tricky bacteria, can break down the antibiotics. It is a weapon the bacteria use against the otherwise lethal onslaught of the antibiotics.

The main approach to outsmarting these bacteria has been to make chemical alterations to the antibiotics that can withstand the destructive enzyme. The newest cephalosporin antibiotics, such as moxalactam and cefotaxime, are highly successful examples of that effort.

Newer penicillins, however, have turned out to be less effective in killing bacteria when altered to defend against the enzyme that can break them down. One of the most intriguing developments in this running battle has been the appearance of new drugs called irreversible beta-lactamase inhibitors. The only job these drugs have is to inactivate the bacterial enzyme—kind of an advance strike force. They have little antibacterial effect themselves, but can pave the way for the use of another highly active penicillin to cure an infection otherwise resistant to this antibiotic.

Two of these inhibitors are clavulanic acid, developed by Beecham Laboratories, and penicillanic acid sulfone, called Sulbactam by its maker, Pfizer Pharmaceuticals Inc. During clinical trials, both have looked quite effective. Clavulanic acid is being combined with amoxicillin (a broad-spectrum penicillin derivative) under the trade name Augmentin, and sulbactam is being combined with ampicillin under the name Sultamicillin. But there is some doubt whether these combination products will be readily accepted by doctors who must prescribe them, since the new-generation antibiotics cefotaxime and moxalactam offer many of these same benefits in a single drug.

Merck Sharp & Dohme has come up with another approach. Researchers there have developed an interesting group of penicillin derivatives called theinamycins. One of these, called imipede, is being tested. It can fight off the destructive bacterial enzymes and still be effective against a broad range of bacteria. One of their main drawbacks is their lack of stability. It has a distressing tendency to break down spontaneously or be degraded by the kidney, although Merck may have licked the problem with a second drug.

The Monobactams: The Backyard Cure

Yet another new group of antibiotics has been christened the monobactams. They are relatives of penicillin, but have a much simpler chemical structure. And the best news is that they are in top form against bacteria that penicillins have trouble killing.

The story behind the discovery of these infection fighters is a fantastic one. All antibiotics are natural products, made by micro-organisms often found in plain old topsoil (dirt). Researchers collect soil samples from all over the world in the hope of chancing upon new microscopic bugs which can produce new antibiotics.

One American drug firm, Squibb Laboratories, sent its workers to check on more than a million soil samples from around the globe. Finally, they found what they were looking for in one of the soil samples. Where had it come from? Practically in the company's own backyard!

Antibiotics of the future are, to some extent, becoming a numbers game. Many of the new drugs have similar uses, and the main difference often is price. Doctors must be very knowledgeable and up-to-date to pick and choose. Making the right choice for a patient can mean a big difference in their treatment.

The New Antibiotics

Penicillins

Brand Name	Generic Name	Advantages
Azlin	azlocillin	Active against *Pseudomonas*
Mezlin	mezlocillin	Active against *Pseudomonas*
Pipracil	piperacillin	Active against *Pseudomonas*
Spectrobid	bacampicillin	Twice daily dosing

Cephalosporins

Claforan	cefotaxime	Better antibacterial activity
Moxam	moxalactam	Better antibacterial activity
Monocid	cefonicid	Long duration
Cefobid	cefoperazone	Long duration
Cefizox	ceftizoxime	Better antibacterial activity
Cefonomil	cefsulodin	Specific for *Pseudomonas*
Rocephin	ceftriaxone	Better antibacterial activity

The New Antibiotics

Zinacef	cefuroxime	None
	ceforanide	Better antibacterial activity
	ceftazidime	Better antibacterial activity
	cefmenoxine	Better antibacterial activity
	cefotetan	Long duration
	cefroxadine	Oral, third generation

Miscellaneous

Augmentin	clavulanic acid + amoxicillin	Inhibits penicillinase
Sultamicillin	sulbactam + ampicillin	Inhibits penicillinase
	imipemide	Better antibacterial activity
Azactam	aztreonam	Better antibacterial activity

14

ANXIETY AND THE
ANTI-VALIUMS

Just about everyone has heard of Valium, the big-selling anti-anxiety drug of recent years. But researchers have also uncovered several related groups of chemicals, including one fascinating group of compounds dubbed the anti-Valiums.

The anti-Valiums do not seem to have any particular effects of their own, except that they specifically block the action of Valium and other drugs in its group, called benzodiazepines. Diazepam, given the trade name Valium by Hoffmann-LaRoche, is the flagship drug of the benzodiazepine class. Benzodiazepines were first developed as antianxiety drugs or tranquilizers, but also turned out to be effective as sleep inducers, anticonvulsants, and muscle relaxers. They continue to be controversial drugs, but like them or not, they are still some of the most widely prescribed medications in America.

Because of this widespread use, the blocking effect of anti-Valium could someday turn out to be a lifesaver. It has been known for years that combining Valium or similar drugs with other depressants such as alcohol can enhance the action of the drug, possibly bringing on severe or fatal side effects. The latest evidence suggests that even taking normal doses of Valium with seemingly innocuous drugs such as birth control pills or the ulcer medication Tagamet (cimetidine) can cause problems.

The reason seems clear: The body's metabolic processes will normally inactivate Valium, if given a chance. But many drugs, including birth control pills and Tagamet, can inhibit this bodily reaction. The result is that Valium's tranquilizing effect is enhanced and prolonged. This can cause unexpected drowsiness, which carries with it the potential for accidents.

What can be done for patients showing signs of oversedation from such a drug combination or overdose? Currently, nothing much, beyond general physical support. In the future, however, the anti-Valiums may be of some help.

On the chemical level, the anti-Valiums are quite similar to Valium. One of the most widely studied of these, bearing the label RO 15–1788, is produced by Hoffmann-LaRoche of Nutley, New Jersey, the same firm that makes Valium. This drug is highly effective in reversing the effects of Valium and other benzodiazepines. It may one day be used to reverse the effects of Valium overdoses, much as naloxone, a narcotic antagonist, reverses the effects of a morphine overdose.

Out of this same research a drug may also eventually come on the market that will help us stay awake and alert without any side effects. One such chemical, 3-hydroxymethyl-beta-carboline, usually called 3-HMC, is already being tested. At low doses it works much like the other anti-Valiums. At high doses, however, it produces a state of quiet but intense wakefulness. The important factor is that this alert state is produced without the undesirable stimulant effects seen with drugs such as amphetamines or caffeine.

Perhaps it was inevitable that research on drugs to take away anxiety also lead to the discovery of other drugs that can actually cause anxiety. What possible use could anxiety-producing drugs be? They are used as research tools, to cause anxiety in laboratory animals so that researchers can figure out more reliable ways of testing drugs to reduce it. One such anxiety-producing product, known as beta-CCE, is already being used for this purpose.

Since the time Valium and its chemical cousins were first introduced to the American public, medical science has learned a great deal more about how fear, anxiety, and depression show up in the chemistry of our bodies. Far from being the vague mental state that we often think of when describing anxiety or depression, there are actually proven chemical differences that take place in your body when you feel those emotions. Scientists have pinpointed those chemicals and have discovered ways to manipulate them with new drugs.

That may or may not be of great medical benefit, depending on how you view the anti-anxiety drugs, better known as tranquilizers. *Without a doubt, turning to drugs to cope with life's problems is no answer.* But scientists have now proven anxiety and depression's biological origins. That means the system is bound to go awry in some people and may require a medical solution to correct the problem. In the vast majority of individuals, anxiety is a familiar and even necessary sensation that carries with it numerous benefits. It is when the system goes haywire, as in so many other diseases, that medical solutions are being sought.

In addition to Valium, other benzodiazepines on the market include; Librium (chlordiazepoxide), Serax (oxazepam), Ativan (lorazepam), Centrax (prazepam), Paxipam (halazepam), Tranxene (chlorazepate), Dalmane (flurazepam), Restoril (temazepam), and the newest entries, Xanax (alpaxolam) and Halcion (triazolam).

For practical purposes, the effects of all these drugs are similar, although Dalmane, Halcion, and Restoril are sold only to produce sleep. There are, however, differences in how long they last and how they are metabolized in the body. With the recent discovery that drugs such as Tagamet and birth control pills can prolong the action of these drugs by inhibiting their metabolism, Ativan (lorazepam) may receive more attention since it is one of the few benzodiazepines inactivated by a different pathway.

Other research is showing that the three actions of Valium—antianxiety, anticonvulsant, and smooth muscle relaxant—can be separated into three different drugs. That means future drug therapy can be aimed more precisely at the problem and eliminate many of the unwanted side effects, although new drugs that may result from this research probably remain years away.

15

THE ARTHRITIS DRUG WARS

The Battle Begins

Aspirin still reigns as the premier arthritis medicine, but the onslaught of a number of new drugs to treat arthritis has caused a heated battle among manufacturers for shares of this huge, and lucrative market. Consumers almost certainly will benefit from the broad new selection of arthritis drugs, but just which product will work best for you can be a highly individual affair.

Although arthritis sufferers are greatly stepping up their spending on arthritis treatment products, there is often little difference in the effectiveness of the available antiarthritis drugs. That is what is now changing, and arthritis sufferers may soon have a different story to tell.

There seems to be a continuous stream of new arthritis drugs in the drug pipeline. Two or more will be added to the list of approved products each year, joining a dozen or so already on the market.

It is not hard to understand the big push by manufacturers to try and capture as big a chunk of the billion-dollar arthritis market as they can. As millions of dollars are devoted to new research, it should be arthritis sufferers who ultimately benefit. Americans are growing older and arthritis is most often associated with aging, so it will be a growing market as well.

Actually, arthritis is a broad term describing nearly a hundred different varieties of the affliction, involving pain and inflammation of the joints. The most common form, osteoarthritis, affects about twenty-five million Americans and is related to aging. About another seven million individuals, primarily young adult women, suffer from a far more severe form of the disease called rheumatoid arthritis. This is believed to be caused by an autoimmune process where the body becomes confused and starts to attack its own joints, thinking they are foreign material. It can cause terrible inflammation of those joints. Normally, the body's immune system is only supposed to fight viruses, bacteria, and other disease producing agents, but in arthritics it somehow goes awry. *Science Digest* magazine described the process like this in an article called "What Is Arthritis?": "Chemicals called prostaglandins start the process by unlocking the door for the immune system's defender cells, called phagocytes. They rush to the scene of the invasion. Some surround and kill the bacteria (for example) and others help clean up the debris. For some unknown reason, the cleanup helpers, called monocytes, can turn into scavengers, releasing enzymes that devour healthy tissues in the joint. Activity from this event attracts other monocytes and the whole process perpetuates itself."

Despite extensive research, the available drugs treat only the symptoms of this painful condition. There is no cure for arthritis, although drugs claiming to bring about arthritis remission are nearing availability.

Drugs available right now fall into two groups: The steroids, such as cortisone, are highly potent hormones with many side effects and are usually used as a last resort. The nonsteroidal, anti-inflammatory agents make up the other group and are among the most widely prescribed drugs in the United States.

In spite of the broadening arthritis drug derby, aspirin is still the standard product most arthritis victims start out with. It is too bad that aspirin lacks the glamor of the prescription products that many people mistakenly believe must work better since a doctor's order is required.

In reality, none of the drugs work particularly well over a long period of time, and even aspirin can cause damage to the stomach lining when taken in the large doses required for effective anti-inflammatory action.

As a result, many arthritis sufferers tend to switch from one drug to another hoping for more relief. That consumer tendency has created fertile ground for new drugs. Profit-conscious manufacturers know that it is easy to overcome consumer loyalty to any particular product since they all fail in the long run.

A Gold Mine for Arthritis Sufferers

Gold . . . many have died in quest of this glittering metal. And many others have been made rich by it. But now a new and far larger group of people stand to benefit from gold—millions of arthritis sufferers.

It is not gold's monetary value that they will be after. It is the metal's chemistry.

A new oral drug, based on gold, shows great promise toward becoming the first product able to support a claim of stopping and even reversing the progress of rheumatoid arthritis. Drug compounds made from gold have been available for many years, but they were all designed to be given by injection, and carried a high risk of toxicity, especially to the kidney.

The new drug, generically called auranofin and sold under the trade name Ridaura, is the first oral, gold antiarthritis agent. Preliminary studies indicate that it has fewer side effects than its injectable cousins, although stomach irritation can be a problem.

If prospects pan out, Ridaura could become one of the more popular in an increasingly crowded field of arthritis drugs, perhaps reaping a gold mine for its manufacturer, SmithKline-Beckman Corporation.

Arthritis sufferers have long been poised for some kind of breakthrough in drug therapy of this widespread disease—something to go beyond simple pain relief or easing of the inflammation. Many have tried but all have come up short.

Two of the most recent contestants have been piroxicam, sold under the trade name Feldene, by Pfizer Pharmaceuticals Inc., and the ill-fated drug benoxaprofen, sold under the trade name Oraflex, by Eli Lilly and Company. In late 1982, Oraflex was pulled from the market indefinitely (probably permanently), pending further study, when it became linked to deaths, especially from heart attacks, and cases of kidney and liver damage.

Feldene—which many people turned to when Oraflex stopped being produced—as well as Oraflex, had shown some early evidence of halting the progress of rheumatoid arthritis, although current thought is that the only real advantage the drugs have is that it need only be taken once a day. That compares to four, five, or six times per day for many other arthritis drugs. The once-a-day, morning or night, advantage could be helpful to forgetful arthritis sufferers. Feldene (piroxicam) was the first of the non-steroidal anti-inflammatory drugs to win approval as a once-a-day arthritis medicine. Pfizer said a twenty-milligram dose can work for twenty-four hours. Although piroxicam is chemically different from other anti-arthritis drugs, it still works the same way by inhibiting the formation of chemicals in the body called prostaglandins, which cause inflammation.

The Oraflex Controversy

Oraflex had a meteoric rise in the United States, and an equally meteoric plunge. In the span of a few months, it was introduced with a flourish by Eli Lilly, achieved spectacular sales to half a million patients; came under attack; and was pulled off the market worldwide by the manufacturer under threat from governments. Arthritis sufferers were promised a medication to use when all else failed, only to have it yanked from their grasp within months of its ceremonial unveiling.

The crusade against Oraflex was led by one of the Ralph Nader organizations, the Health Research Group, which is frequently biting at the heels of the FDA and the drug industry; often with good reason.

When reports in a British medical journal linked benoxaprofen (Oraflex) to kidney and liver damage, as well as many deaths in elderly patients, the group asked the FDA to take it off the market. The drug had been available in England under the trade name Opren for about two years before it was approved in the United States.

The possibility of liver damage has not been limited to just benoxaprofen, but has also been linked to other non-steroidal anti-inflammatory drugs over the years. This has led to a label change on these drugs warning of possible liver toxicity.

In one particularly acrid confrontation over Oraflex, an Eli Lilly official, Dr. Ian Shedden, and Health Research Group Director Dr. Sidney Wolfe, squared off on public television's *MacNeil-Lehrer Report.* Shedden called the charges against his company's drug "a gross overreaction to the situation." Asked why Oraflex is a useful drug, Shedden said, ". . . because arthritis is a very difficult disease to treat. There are a number of drugs available for its management, but at any point in time, approximately thirty percent of all patients suffering from arthritis are taking no prescription medication at all. No drug suits everybody. Each drug provides something for everybody. Some drugs provide a lot for a small number of people. Oraflex clearly is an important introduction in a largely unsatisfied market."

Wolfe called Lilly's denial of any clear link between Oraflex and the reported deaths "a reckless, irresponsible kind of statement. . . . For Eli Lilly to say that there's no evidence that Oraflex causes death, no causal relationship, is like the Tobacco Institute saying, as they do today, that there's no evidence of causal relationship linking cigarettes with lung cancer."

Several months after the televised confrontation, the Health Research Group was calling for criminal prosecution of the Eli Lilly Company for allegedly withholding evidence that Oraflex contributed to deaths and liver and kidney damage. But the FDA admits it failed to evaluate all the data Lilly provided, using the excuse that Lilly failed to draw these toxic effects to the agency's attention.

Even before the main part of the controversy broke, there were accusations that Eli Lilly's advertising claims for the drug were far overblown, and that Oraflex was misrepresented in press releases sent to newspapers and television stations all over the country. The FDA later chastised Lilly for the way the Oraflex publicity was handled. The drug was portrayed as a major new development, different from what was already available (the same type of claim often made by drug companies in a highly competitive field) when that was not quite the case.

All the publicity prompted by Lilly's efforts also led many arthritis sufferers to pressure physicians into prescribing the new drug—something more than one doctor came to resent. Was that improper? Arthritis expert Dr. Israeli Jaffe had this to say on *The MacNeil-Lehrer Report:* "For many of us who practice rheumatic diseases alone, the phone scarcely stopped ringing for a day or two after that press conference (held by Lilly). Not only did they ask for the drug but they were resentful that we hadn't given it to them sooner."

Jaffe went on to say: "I feel very strongly that the public has a right to know when significant breakthroughs are made in medical research. Firstly, they're vitally concerned and secondly, they've paid for this. They've paid for it at the local pharmacy when they buy the drug and they pay for it with their tax dollars which supports much of the research. And I think that if and when there are breakthroughs—and we know what a breakthrough drug is—it should be made a media event in short order. When a new drug comes along which may be better in certain respects than others and indeed may be worse in other respects, I think the public should be made aware of its existence but in a low-key fashion appropriate to the contribution of the drug at the point in time that it is introduced. I think ethical pharmaceuticals, drugs that are available by prescription, not over-the-counter, should not be introduced like toothpaste and breakfast cereal. It's far too serious a matter."

Says Jaffe about arthritis sufferers: "They're always looking for a panacea elsewhere, largely because we in this specialty have been failures in terms of really good drug therapy. Our progress has been very slow. So that what happens is it's a yo-yo phenomenon. Their spirits get buoyed up by publicity, they get the drug, they badger the physicians for it, and many wind up being disappointed."

ACTIVITY AND SIDE EFFECTS

Feldene, as well as Oraflex, has some significant side effects. Feldene can produce stomach discomfort and ulcers, as well as dizziness and changes in blood and kidney functions. Oraflex was able to sidestep the ulcer problem but also made people highly sensitive to light and caused some people's fingernails to separate from the skin. Exposure to sunlight while taking Oraflex could cause rash and other skin reactions. One British study also linked the use of Oraflex to increased hair growth in all areas of the body in both men and women.

Current and Coming Arthritis Drugs

The king of the arthritis drug mountain has been a drug called Motrin (ibuprofen), made by The Upjohn Company. It has recently been approved as a general pain reliever. (The same drug made by another company is called Rufen.) But with plenty of other climbers, that is changing. Competitors that are being vigorously marketed include Feldene (made by Pfizer Pharmaceuticals), Naprosyn (made by Syntex Laboratories Inc.), Clinoril and Indocin (both made by Merck Sharp & Dohme), Nalfon (Eli Lilly), Tolectin (Johnson & Johnson), and Meclomen (Warner-Lambert Company).

With the many new nonsteroidal anti-inflammatory drugs (NSAIDs) on the market, doctors are having to choose among the many subtle differences that the drugs offer. They accomplish roughly the same end, but with minor variations in how they get there. For example, the time it takes for the drug to reach peak levels in the blood can vary among the NSAIDs. According to a comparison appearing in *Modern Medicine,* Tolectin takes from half an hour to an hour, Clinoril from two to four hours, Feldene from three to five hours, Meclomen from half an hour to an hour, and Nalfon, Motrin, and Rufen from one to two hours. The combinations of possible side effects are numerous, and often include rash, itching, stomach upset, diarrhea, dizziness, headache, drowsiness, blurred vision, and a ringing in the ears known as tinnitus.

Besides the gold-based drug Ridaura, other arthritis products waiting in the wings include Cinopal (Lederle Laboratories), Rengasil (Ciba-Geigy Corporation), Ridamyl (Roche Laboratories), and Flenac (Norwich-Eaton Pharmaceuticals), Maxicam (Warner-Lambert), Orudis (Ives), Ultradol (Ayerst), and Ciradol (Wyeth).

The chemical onslaught against arthritis has been accelerating, in part because medical science is getting closer to a complete understanding of the disease. But in large measure, many of the new drugs still miss their mark because the complex mechanisms of arthritis remain elusive.

The real force behind all these products is the size and, more importantly, the consistency of the market. Many of the seven million rheumatoid arthritis victims develop the disease in their thirties and forties and live normal lifetimes.

Also among the promising findings is a three-drug combination said to work against very severe arthritis. Azathioprine and cyclophosphamide, both drugs that have an effect on the body's natural immune system, and hydroxychloroquine, a malaria drug, were reported to be the three drugs producing the positive results in one small experiment. A report on this episode in the *Journal of the American Medical Association (JAMA)* said several patients achieved complete remission of their advanced rheumatoid arthritis with this combination of drugs.

By now arthritis patients have accepted the fact that there is no cure for their disease and that they may have to take drugs for many years to relieve the symptoms. One can only hope that medicine makes even greater strides in the future in understanding what causes arthritis, and that a cure may someday be possible.

16

ARTIFICIAL BLOOD CAN WORK

The term "red-blooded" is not yet in danger of becoming obsolete, but medical science is moving in that direction. Call it manmade, artificial, or fake blood, however you say it, Fluosol is not the real thing and does not look like the real thing (it is not red), but it is already saving lives. Blood shortages and toxic reactions to transfusions could one day become a thing of the past.

Green Cross, a giant drug concern in Japan, makes the only widely available artificial blood product. Its full name is Fluosol-DA and it is a mixture of two different substances called fluorocarbons —perfluorodecalin and perfluorotripropylamine. This combination results in a stable substance that is rapidly eliminated from the body through the lungs. Since these chemicals are not metabolized by the body, it was important to find something that would not stick around inside the patient for long periods of time.

Impressive results in animal studies led to human testing, beginning in Japan in 1979. Those ongoing studies have also proven the substance to be effective, although approval was slow in coming in Japan and the drug company ran into trouble at one point for apparently conducting tests without government approval. The

Alpha-Therapeutic Corporation, a North American subsidiary of Green Cross, has been conducting further independent studies of the artificial blood in the United States and Canada.

In cases where Fluosol has been used in the United States the results were encouraging. Some of the patients were dangerously anemic and had refused traditional blood transfusions because of religious beliefs. With artificial blood there was a significant improvement in the oxygen available to their tissues and none of them suffered significant adverse effects.

Despite these encouraging initial tests, it is important to keep in mind that artificial blood is not a complete blood replacement. The only use these fluorocarbons really have is to carry large amounts of oxygen. Unlike real blood, they do not have the essential proteins such as antibodies to fight infection, and they lack clotting factors to prevent bleeding.

That means the uses of artificial blood will be limited to a few specific applications, but those are certainly significant. If the safety of Fluosol is verified by large clinical studies, this, or something similar to it, may be available as a temporary treatment for patients with an inadequate blood supply. New and improved artificial blood products are already being worked on. Although it will not totally replace natural blood, Fluosol's oxygen-carrying ability can be life-saving.

The other efforts to come up with artificial blood or blood substitutes have also been showing progress. Synthetic red blood cells that may be even better than Fluosol because they carry more oxygen, are metabolized by the system, and cause no immune reactions are being pursued. And military doctors in the United States have been working on a hemoglobin-based powder that, when mixed in water, can serve to carry oxygen through the body in an emergency.

Every year, people die because of reactions to the blood they received in a transfusion, because of an inadvertent transfer of hepatitis, or because their religion forbids them to receive blood.

What is more important, there seems to be a constant shortage of real blood, despite periodic pleas from the Red Cross for more donors.

Further advances in artificial blood could make these problems disappear. Manmade blood is stable, has universal utility, and is good for months or even years if frozen. Donated blood must be refrigerated and still goes bad in about twenty-one days. Artificial blood can be given to people with any blood type without delays for cross-matching. In an emergency, this feature could save many lives.

17

ASPIRIN: A TABLET A DAY MAY KEEP MORE THAN HEADACHES AWAY

Almost since its discovery nearly a century ago, aspirin has been the single most widely used drug in the world. It is potent stuff, and some people like to say that the federal government would never let it on the market if it came up for approval under today's strict and lengthy drug approval process. That is an intriguing thought, but there is probably little truth to the claim.

Aspirin is a remarkably safe drug—and remember that it *is* a drug—within limits, and when used as a pain reliever or as a fever reducer.

What is astounding about aspirin is the incredible list of other benefits that medical science is now turning up for this ubiquitous medication. Although the American public inevitably associates aspirin with headaches, it now appears that aspirin may help prevent some far more serious disorders. These include heart attacks, strokes, the plugging of arteries transplanted during coronary bypass surgery, cataracts, gallstones, and even some kinds of cancer. Some doctors are now hedging their bets by taking a daily dose of aspirin themselves, in case there turns out to be more to aspirin than meets the eye.

Aspirin's roots go way back. Salicin, a natural chemical cousin of aspirin that is found in the bark of certain willow and poplar trees, was prescribed for pain over two thousand years ago. Little did these ancient physicians know what they were on to.

But in its pure form, this chemical is far too irritating for people to take. It was not until the 1890s that a chemical company in Germany found an answer. The company, named Bayer, found that a derivative, acetylsalicylic acid, was both tolerable and effective. When it hit the market in 1899, the company gave this white crystalline powder a name: Aspirin.

As the drug quickly caught on in the United States, aspirin became the generic name. Today it is estimated that Americans swallow about ninety million of the little white pills every day. Despite plenty of would-be competitors developed over the years, aspirin remains the prototype of the non-narcotic pain reliever (analgesic). It is also the main treatment for rheumatoid arthritis, a serious form of that disease, even though many new and promising arthritis drugs have either become available or will soon be in the United States (See Chapter 15, *The Arthritis Drug Wars*).

Walk into a drugstore and you will encounter aspirin in various forms at just about every turn. There are some forty thousand OTC drug products in the United States today that contain aspirin.

The details of just how aspirin works mysteriously evaded researchers until 1971 when they finally discovered that aspirin blocks the formation of chemicals called prostaglandins, which are found throughout your body. These chemicals have been linked to a wide variety of effects in the body, including pain, inflammation, production of a coating that protects the stomach from its own acid, and also an early step in blood clotting called platelet aggregation or simply clumping. Some of aspirin's effects are still not fully understood, however.

It is the effect on blood clotting that is getting the most attention. Why? Because stopping the small blood cells called platelets from clumping can help prevent strokes and heart attacks. Here is how it works.

Technically, aspirin is able to prevent the formation of prostaglandins in the body by short-circuiting an enzyme that is crucial to the process. This enzyme is called cyclooxygenase. An indirect result of this activity prevents the formation of other chemicals called thromboxanes, which are the ultimate cause of platelet clumping.

Since the effect of the aspirin on this enzyme is irreversible, and the body takes several days to produce more of the enzyme, a single dose of aspirin can prevent clumping for the entire lifetime of the small platelet blood cells, which is anywhere from seven to ten days. That means large and frequent doses of aspirin are not needed to achieve this important effect. In fact, as little as one aspirin tablet—usually 325 milligrams—will inhibit clumping for forty-eight hours.

So What?

The obvious question about all of this complicated biochemistry is whether there is any practical medical benefit to these effects of aspirin.

For preventing strokes, the answer is almost certainly Yes, with studies to prove it. People who took four aspirin daily in one study were highly successful in decreasing the number of strokes they suffered. There is even evidence that still better results could be achieved with *lower* doses of aspirin.

Aspirin's ability to prevent heart attacks is less clear-cut, but still seems to exist. Since only some heart attacks are caused by blood clots, there's been a problem in finding out for sure because of the lack of good research data. For some reason, several of the studies only looked at the benefits of aspirin in preventing *second* heart attacks in patients who survived a first. Aspirin does seem to significantly reduce the chances of a second attack and a recent study showed it is as good as the potent anticoagulants (blood thinners) used more commonly today. It stands to reason that the same might apply for preventing first heart attacks as well, and since aspirin is so safe it could be used before one could justify the use of an anticoagulant.

Unfortunately, aspirin's benefits follow sexual lines. The most dramatic clinical benefits seem to involve men and not women. Why this happens is not clear to scientists yet, but it may have something to do with how aspirin affects blood clots that do form— a process that can differ between sexes.

The experimental evidence is still hazy, but the potential benefits, and the fact that aspirin is cheap, relatively safe, and readily available, have caused lots of people to start looking at aspirin in new ways, including as a preventative treatment.

Another approach being used to prevent the formation of blood clots, especially after surgery, is to combine aspirin with a drug called dipyridamole. This drug, marketed under the trade name Persantine, seems to enhance the beneficial effects of the aspirin. In patients undergoing coronary bypass surgery, this combination can prolong the time the bypass grafts remain free of clots, which is a common problem after this increasingly common operation.

The First Drug for Cataracts?

There's also much excitement that aspirin will turn out to be the first drug able to prevent the onset of cataracts. This eye disease, which can progress to blindness, is common in diabetics and the elderly.

But amazingly, research has suggested that simply taking four aspirin daily could delay the development of cataracts for several years. The sad part of this discovery is that aspirin does not seem able to reverse cataracts once they have formed. New studies are trying to find out more about aspirin's preventative powers over cataracts.

Even some forms of cancer, with all its dumbfounding properties, may prove susceptible to little old aspirin. Laboratory studies are showing evidence that aspirin can slow the progress of one kind of liver cancer in animals, as well as the invasion of cancer into bone and other tissues.

Still another feather in aspirin's hat is its purported ability to block the formation of gallstones. Evidence is sketchy but highly suggestive that regular aspirin doses can stop the gallbladder from secreting excess mucin that can cause the stones to form.

Should We All Become Aspirin Junkies?

If aspirin is so great, why don't we all start gobbling it up every day? It may be a certified miracle drug, but it would not be wise to say that everyone should start taking aspirin every day in hopes of warding off a variety of ills. Medical experts do *not* recommend such an approach. Aspirin is a powerful drug, despite its easy availability without a prescription, and its use shouldn't be taken lightly.

Since aspirin is an acid, it can wreak havoc with the stomach, and people with ulcers should avoid it. Aspirin's effects on blood platelets is usually beneficial, but can also be harmful by slowing down clotting and inducing excess bleeding. Recent research suggests this can be a particular problem for pregnant women.

Taking aspirin in combination with other drugs can cause problems. Taken together with oral products for diabetes or anticoagulants, aspirin can enhance the effects of these drugs and result in a serious reaction.

Aspirin can even be fatal, particularly in children whose bodies cannot compensate for a sudden influx of acid in the blood from an aspirin overdose: In 1965, aspirin accounted for twenty-five percent of child poisonings in the United States. That figure has dropped to only about four percent today, mostly because of the law requiring child-proof containers for aspirin products, but aspirin is still a leading cause of poisoning. Adults are not immune either to the potentially toxic effects of large aspirin doses, and excess aspirin use has even been linked to the death of recluse billionaire Howard Hughes.

The Reye's Syndrome Controversy

On the negative side, there is a rare but extremely dangerous disorder in children that has been linked to the use of aspirin. The disorder, Reye's syndrome, named after the Australian doctor who discovered it, is fatal twenty to thirty percent of the time, yet it remains unexplained. It strikes youngsters under the age of fifteen after a viral illness such as the flu or chickenpox. The symptoms include vomiting, delirium, and weakness followed by coma and brain swelling that must be treated to prevent brain damage or death.

No one knows what causes Reye's syndrome, nor how to cure it, but some evidence points to aspirin as the culprit since most of the victims took the drug. Coincidence? The manufacturers of aspirin say it is, and that children running a fever would be expected to receive aspirin. Even so, the numbers point the other direction. About ninety-six percent of Reye's syndrome victims took aspirin for their flu or chickenpox. At the same time, only sixty-two percent of the children who did not develop the syndrome took aspirin for their flu or chickenpox.

With some prodding from consumer and medical groups, the FDA has ordered that warning labels be placed on aspirin and aspirin-containing products, and that doctors, pharmacists, and parents be advised of the potential risks involving aspirin and Reye's syndrome.

Perhaps the message coming out of this controversy is that *lowering a fever with drugs, aspirin, or otherwise, may not always be the right thing to do.* Few people realize that fever is a natural bodily defense used to defeat an invading organism. Shortcircuiting this defense, by taking aspirin, could actually prevent your body from adequately defending itself.

With these new discoveries, aspirin seems certain to hold its place as the oldest miracle of modern medicine. It is proving that the newest drug is not always the best.

18

ASTHMA DRUGS: BECOMING MORE SELECTIVE

Fighting asthma attacks with drugs has always been a rather tricky business. Ideally, the drug should affect only the bronchial muscle (the so-called smooth or involuntary muscle) and nothing else. But asthma drugs also affect the heart, causing all kinds of potentially serious complications.

Slowly, however, the selectivity of asthma drugs is being improved as some new drugs have reached the market, with still others on the way. They are more selective, which is to say they affect mostly the bronchial smooth muscle, they act quicker, last longer, and cause fewer side effects.

But even the new ones, with all these advantages, are still far from perfect, and side effects remain distressingly frequent. Albuterol, for example, which was approved for prescription use in the United States in 1981 as an inhalant, and later as a tablet, causes twenty percent of the people who take it to develop nervous tremors. Another seven percent of users experience headaches, and five percent develop heart palpitations. As a result, this, and similar drugs, should be used cautiously by people with high blood pressure, heart disease, or diabetes.

Sterling Drug Inc. has sought government approval for another new asthma drug called Tornalate—the company's brand name for bitolterol. Sterling says its aerosol bronchodilator will help in the prevention and treatment of bronchial asthma and other disorders involving constriction of the bronchial airways, including exercise-induced bronchospasm. The firm also claims the drug works mainly on the lungs, thereby minimizing many of the side effects seen with similar products. The clinical trials for Tornalate, which Sterling claimed were the most extensive ever conducted for an aerosol bronchodilator, have apparently shown it works quickly, and is well tolerated.

Left untreated, asthma can be a very debilitating disorder, with repeated and unpredictable attacks of coughing, difficulty in breathing, and wheezing. The goal of drug therapy is to prevent or reverse the uncomfortable and possibly life-threatening effects of an attack.

About half of all individuals with asthma get it before the age of ten, and eighty percent will have developed it by age thirty. The attacks characteristic of asthma can last a few minutes or several days. The availability of several nonprescription asthma medications presents some dangers for people who try to self-diagnose their problem as asthma. The OTC asthma, or bronchodilator products should never be used unless a physician has already diagnosed the problem as being asthma. It could very well be something entirely different that could be made even worse by using the asthma drugs.

Even when the problem is definitely asthma, the American Pharmaceutical Association's *Handbook of Nonprescription Drugs* says the most common over-the-counter asthma products are only moderately effective even when properly used (improper use is a major problem with inhalers), and are possibly less safe than the asthma medications only available by prescription.

The new asthma drugs available by prescription belong to a class called beta-2 agonists (opposite of antagonist) which stimulate a particular type of nerve, causing a relaxation of the bronchial muscles. Earlier bronchodilators, such as epinephrine and isoproterenol, were not as selective and had a greater effect on the heart and brain. Albuterol also seems to have an edge over some other beta-2 agonists such as metaproterenol (Alupent, Metaprel) and terbutaline (Brethine, Bricanyl), in that it has fewer side effects.

When albuterol was approved it quickly became the most widely prescribed bronchodilator. It is sold under the brand names Ventolin and Proventil. In tablet form, albuterol has been shown to improve the functioning of the lung in an asthmatic within thirty minutes of taking the drug, although the effect lasts only about six or eight hours. The drug would have to be taken some three or four times daily.

Although the selectivity of the newer drugs is still only relatively better than the old, how the drug is given can also have an effect on selectivity. When inhaled, instead of given in pill form, the drug stays where it is supposed to be—in the lung—and does not travel as easily to other parts of the system. Another long-time concern about the buildup of a resistance to the asthma medications remains unanswered and under investigation.

The aerosols are most often used when an asthma attack starts, with the effects lasting varying lengths of time. Sterling claims Tornalate will have a prolonged effect, although just how long is not certain.

Beware also that these new asthma drugs may interact with other medications, producing unwanted results. For example, albuterol's effects would be completely blocked if the individual is also taking a heart drug known as a beta blocker for such ailments as hypertension or angina. Albuterol should also be avoided by people who are taking antidepressant medications because of the likelihood the drug interaction will increase toxicity.

19

CAFFEINE OR
NO CAFFEINE?

Asked to name the most widely consumed drug in the world, most people would probably say aspirin. That is a good guess, but aspirin actually runs a poor second. Caffeine is the most extensively used drug.

Far from being the innocuous stimulant most people assume, caffeine is a powerful drug with more evidence all the time suggesting it can do plenty to harm you. Some of caffeine's long-recognized effects on the body include: constriction of blood vessels, increased stomach acid and urine production (hence the frequent trips to the bathroom), relaxation of bronchial muscles, and stimulation of heart contractions.

But until recently, the reasons why caffeine caused these things to happen remained unclear. It is now believed that many of caffeine's effects can be explained by how it inhibits the action of a body chemical called adenosine.

Under normal circumstances, adenosine blocks the transmission of certain nerve impulses in the brain and elsewhere. Thus, as caffeine removes this natural roadblock, the nerve impulses have a clear path and you feel the stimulant effect. If you regularly consume lots of caffeine, your body may try to compensate by producing more adenosine to counteract its effects.

That physiological change is responsible for the feeling of being hooked that high caffeine doses can create. Do not kid yourself, there is a genuine physical dependency on the stuff.

Cutting out your caffeine intake suddenly can cause equally real withdrawal symptoms. The reason is that your body continues to compensate even after you stop consuming caffeine. The symptoms of this caffeine withdrawal—which disappear after a short time—can include headaches, irritability, and weakness.

The Emergence of Caffeinism

Excess caffeine intake—caffeinism—is characterized by rapid, shallow breathing, nervousness, mood changes, tremors, and heart palpitations.

Victims and doctors alike can be fooled into thinking these symptoms point to another disease of some kind. People often fail to recognize all of the sources they may be getting caffeine from, which added together can amount to toxic levels. Pure caffeine is a potent substance and possibly fatal at a dose of about ten grams. Fortunately, your body quickly disposes of caffeine and such a large dose could not be ingested from normal sources.

Where does most of your caffeine intake come from? Coffee provides the greatest bulk of it, but it is not the only source. Soft drinks, teas, and chocolate are three other suppliers.

Another major source are common drugstore products, including pain relievers such as Anacin, Cope, and Excedrin, stay-awake drugs such as No-doz and Vivarin, and many nonprescription diet aids such as Dexatrim and Ayds.

Caffeine doesn't just happen to be in many of these drug products. Some contain it naturally, but in others the manufacturers put it there precisely to make use of the known effects of the drug. Since caffeine interferes with sleep, it's a natural for products designed to keep you awake and alert.

In headache preparations, the caffeine is there to constrict the blood vessels in your head (one effect it probably does not have). It's the dilation of those vessels that may be causing the ache.

Cola-type soft drinks contain some caffeine naturally from the kola nut, but they are often supplemented with even more in order to provide the advertised lift. The origins of doing so may be traced back to the days when cocaine was actually an ingredient in one cola drink.

Surprisingly, it was not until mid-1982, when 7-Up started pushing its product as better because it had no caffeine, that the multibillion-dollar soft-drink industry differentiated between caffeine and no caffeine. Coffee makers did it years ago. Suddenly, caffeine joined a long list of other substances the public discovered could be hazardous to your health.

Still, there is an undeniably pleasant stimulant effect that many people like, or need, particularly to get going in the morning. Its natural origins, long history of use, and the long-time perception that it cannot really hurt you, have landed caffeine on the federal government's list of food additives classified as "generally recognized as safe," which carries the bureaucratic acronym GRAS. It means that caffeine is exempt from most regulatory tests required of new additives and, until recently, from public concern about its safety.

The Evidence: How Conclusive?

The evidence against caffeine in some areas is not all that conclusive. The effects have been studied and restudied but no one yet knows precisely what hazards caffeine poses beyond the relatively mild withdrawal syndrome. The most feared hazards are probably the most questionable—birth defects, heart disease, cancer, and the worsening of fibrocystic breast disease in women.

Since pregnant women consume much caffeine along with everybody else, birth defects are one of the greatest concerns. Studies with rats are what established this link in the first place, but that is far from conclusive since many drugs, including aspirin, can cause birth defects in rats but not in humans. The results of one Harvard University study, published in the *New England Journal of Medicine,* suggested that caffeine consumption has a minimal effect, if any, on the outcome of a pregnancy. Since coffee drinkers can also be smokers, researchers find it hard to separate the effects of nicotine from those of caffeine. Nevertheless, the FDA has warned against caffeine consumption by pregnant women because of the harmful effects noted in animal studies in the laboratory.

Caffeine is probably no more dangerous than most of the other natural chemicals you ingest every day, but it can nonetheless cause problems. Caution would dictate minimizing or eliminating as much caffeine consumption as possible.

20

CANCER: A CHINK
IN THE ARMOR

The War Drags On

Remember the beginnings of the great war on cancer declared by President Nixon back in the late 1960s? People thought of it as another race to the moon, expecting a cure within a few years once federal money was behind the battle. When the battle troops floundered, and the hope for a cure faded, federal support for cancer research slowed. The business sector had never really even joined the fray. People started thinking cancer would never be licked.

Free enterprise was not particularly kind to cancer victims when it came to going out on a financial limb to find effective anticancer drugs. What America failed to realize at the beginning was that cancer is not a single disease—no more than the term "American" indicates a common ancestry.

Cancer is a family of diseases, and a tremendously large family at that. The term lung cancer, for example, is thrown around frequently, but it hardly pinpoints the type of cancer involved. There are many cancers that can befall lung tissue.

This multiplicity of cancers has proven a formidable foe. Chemotherapy, the use of chemicals or drugs to treat cancer, has only been able to skirt the edges. Still, with ten million cancer victims living in the United States today, the pursuit of a "magic bullet" or miracle cure against the killer disease continues to have a big emotional draw within the medical and pharmaceutical fields. It is an expensive search and the findings have not been particularly astounding, so many profit-minded drug companies have only dabbled in cancer drugs.

Since no single drug has yet been found to have broad usefulness against many types of cancer, it remains, economically, a market of many little drugs. Each product must be able to target specific types of cancer cells.

In spite of the difficulties, some cancers are being cured. Nearly a third of the 835,000 new cancer victims each year can be cured with nothing more than surgery or radiation. These curable cancers have not usually spread very far and thus can be more easily treated. Early detection is the key. Once cancer has spread (metastasized), treatment gets tougher.

Now even widespread cancers are being successfully treated with drugs that are themselves undergoing steady improvement. It has not always been the case, but most advanced cancers are now treated with some type of drug. Cancer research is building steam again.

Of more than a million chemical combinations tested for anticancer value over the last twenty-five years, only about forty turned out to have any use against human cancers. There still are not any miracle drugs, but at least drug companies seem finally to be drawn into the cancer field. Cancer drugs are selling. The leader has been the Bristol-Myers Company, which markets several of the best-selling anticancer products.

With the alternative often being death, rules for testing new drugs in cancer victims are less strict than for other diseases. Cancer victims have roughly a thirty percent chance of receiving something useful in these tests, but often the biggest accomplishment is paving the way for somebody else's life to be saved.

DRUG INDUCED CURES NOW POSSIBLE

With some types of cancer, it is now reasonable to expect that a drug may actually produce a cure. The number of cancer patients cured by chemotherapy quadrupled from about ten thousand in 1972 to over forty thousand in 1982.

The list of cancer types that will succumb to drug therapy is also growing. Cures are now expected fifty to eighty percent of the time in these types of cancer: leukemia, Hodgkin's disease, diffuse histiocytic lymphoma, testicular cancer, choriocarcinoma, Wilms' tumor, Ewing's tumor, embryonal rhabdomyosarcoma, and Burkitt's lymphoma.

But a major problem of anticancer drugs is still their poor aim. They are not able to pick out the exact cancer cells to attack. That is not surprising since, biochemically, cancer cells are not much different than normal cells. Most cancer drugs in the past were merely instructed to attack the cells that divided most rapidly. That usually got the cancer, but also damaged bone marrow, hair cells, and cells lining the mouth, stomach, and intestine.

New and promising ideas to improve the aim of these cancer drugs are being investigated.

Fighting Cancer with Antibodies

Antibodies, armed with microscopic weapons designed specifically to attack a cancerous tumor, are one of the most intriguing possibilities in an emerging branch of medical technology—monoclonal antibodies. They are antibodies that scientists hope will one day be used to effectively detect and fight cancer.

If other cancer treatments are considered the shotgun approach, then the monoclonal antibodies would be the rifle-shot approach. Antibodies in general are natural substances that can recognize and bind to specific targets in the body, called antigens. An ideal anticancer antibody would recognize an antigen found only in a particular cancer tumor. But there do not seem to be any such antigens found exclusively in cancer tumors.

The next best thing is an antigen found in tumors more often than elsewhere. But medicine is again stymied because not all tumors of a given type have the same antigens, meaning that patients with the same cancer could not be treated with the same antibody.

Another problem: For an antibody to be useful against cancer, one that specifically reacts with a tumor would be needed, and it would have to be available in large amounts and in a pure form. It might seem relatively simple to isolate the cell making the antibody you want, grow lots of those cells in a lab culture, and collect the antibody the cells produce. The problem is that spleen cells, where the antibodies are produced, do not grow well in artificial systems.

The solution was the discovery of hybridomas. A hybridoma is the result of fusing a normal cell with one that will grow continuously in a lab culture. In practice, this requires mixing spleen cells with cells called myeloma cells. But that is not easy either. Only one in every two hundred thousand spleen cells will form a hybridoma, and even then you must screen for the hybrids that produce the one antibody you are looking for.

It is tedious, but the result of a successful experiment is an immortal clone that will produce virtually unlimited amounts of the specific antibody desired.

Some of the first clinical work with monoclonal antibodies has focused on early detection of cancer, since the earlier cancer is discovered the more likely a cure becomes. Scientists have tried screening blood samples for tumor antigens. Antibodies, linked with special chemicals, have also been combined with new X-ray technology to try and improve the accuracy of this technique. So far, however, it has not been very successful.

The idea of linking monoclonal antibodies with cell-killing agents is another course, and early work has focused on a cell toxin from castor beans called ricin. Researchers have shown that an antibody-ricin duo can kill the abnormal blood cells characteristic of leukemia in mice without harming normal cells. Should this also work in humans, a highly effective, fairly nontoxic treatment for leukemia could become available.

Antibodies alone can also stimulate natural immune responses in the body that kill tumor cells. This has been tried in patients with lymphoma—with some success, but the antibodies must be made specifically for each individual patient, and the slow, tedious procedure needed to develop monoclonal antibodies makes widespread use of this method unlikely.

There are concerns about toxicity in the use of monoclonal antibodies. Human antibodies are not yet available, and antibodies from mouse cells have been used instead. The repeated use of these foreign proteins in human patients could lead to severe allergic reactions. This has spawned a major effort to develop human monoclonal antibodies.

Scientists may find that a widely usable product will require mixtures of monoclonal antibodies and that will tend to increase the risk of attacks on normal cells. Dramatic strides have been made in the 1970s since the discovery of monoclonal antibodies, but useful anticancer products remain years away.

Genetic engineering, nevertheless, may help accelerate the assault on cancer more than anything else has in recent years. By gene splicing's super-sophisticated techniques, cancer researchers will be able to extract from our own genes the natural codes for fighting cancer. It will give them the tools to finally pinpoint causes of the disease and find ways to prevent it, including vaccines against cancer.

Shedding Light on the Matter: Lasers and Drugs Against Cancer

New drugs that make cancer cells sensitive to light are also offering hope of improved selectivity. A drug called hematoporphyrin that seems to collect in tumor cells and not in normal cells can cause the light sensitivity.

In this space-aged technique, the next step is to beam a special type of laser light into the tumor. The light energizes the drug which then destroys the cancerous cells. Since the normal cells have captured little of the drug, they are spared.

The hematoporphyrin itself seems to have few side effects. Tests in 150 patients with cancer using this photoradiation technique have reduced tumors by fifty percent or more in most patients. Some actually seemed to be cured.

Photoradiation can be teamed up with other types of cancer therapy. It is a new method that may be able to treat some types of cancer once considered hopeless. Although only discovered in the late 1970s, the light treatment is already being used around the world.

Another dynamic anticancer duo may be drugs and X rays. A curious drug called misonidazole can apparently increase the sensitivity of tumors to X rays, much as the other drug heightens light sensitivity. That is important because most tumors have low susceptibility to X rays because of an inadequate oxygen supply. Misonidazole, once activated by the X rays, then turns and destroys the tumor cells, with few additional effects on normal cells.

Magnetic Microspheres

Eli Lilly Company is developing another drug delivery system—the magnetic microsphere method. An anti-cancer drug is formulated into microscopic spheres containing iron which are then injected into the patient. A magnetic field focused over the tumor then draws the spheres to the cancer site. The method seems to show better results at a lower drug dose and with fewer side effects.

New Avenues of Approach

The variety of conventional cancer drugs in use, being tested, or under development is far too lengthy to cover in detail. A few of the biggest sellers, according to *The New York Times,* are Platinol, Cytoxan, Blenoxane, and Mutamycin, all sold by Bristol-Myers; Adriamycin marketed by Adria Laboratories; Methotrexate, marketed by American Cynamid; and Oncovin and Velban marketed by Eli Lilly.

Most anticancer drugs work by interrupting the ability of cancer cells to divide. If they cannot divide, they cannot grow. However, the drugs are limited in their ability to go very far with this by their toxic effects on normal cells. Drug combinations with varying dosages and timing are sometimes used to get the best kill results with minimum side effects.

Using two or more drugs in sequence (rather than together) is another concept that has turned up positive results. Using the drug methotrexate first, for example, can set up the cancer cells for a subsequent kill by another drug called 5-fluorouracil.

A problem is that most of the existing drugs are related to one another in some way, and therefore have similar side effects. The idea now is to find something with fewer side effects. There have been some successes, but there may be a brighter future in taking entirely new approaches. There are already a few unique new products worth mentioning.

A drug called leuprolide shows promise against prostatic cancer. It works by blocking the release of hormones needed by these cancer cells to survive. Studies have shown a remission rate of 50 percent, with few side effects. One cannot be sure whether this really represents a cure since most tumors can reappear unless remission is maintained for five years.

Bimolane, a drug discovered in China, also looks useful against some kinds of cancer. Given orally, bimolane has been reported to produce regression of some tumors such as Hodgkin's disease and cancer of the vulva. Toxic effects included mild intestinal effects and a slight decrease in white blood cells. Further studies in the United States will be necessary before a better evaluation of this drug can be made.

One unique new product that finally achieved FDA approval is streptozocin. (Also see Chapter 8, *Orphan Drugs Are Up for Adoption.*) To be sold as Zanosar by Upjohn, this product specifically attacks cells in the pancreas called islet cells, which normally produce insulin but occasionally become cancerous. Although damaging to the kidneys and toxic to normal islet cells as well as the cancerous ones, this drug is the best thing available for those few people who get pancreatic cancer.

A DRUG TO EASE SIDE EFFECTS

As already noted, most of the anticancer drugs carry with them severe side effects, including nausea and vomiting. Much attention is now being focused on separate drugs to ease those side effects.

One successful product deserving mention is metoclopramide, sold as Reglan by the A. H. Robins Company. The drug has no use against cancer per se, except as a highly effective antivomiting agent to make it easier for people to take the other drugs that do attack the cancer. Reglan seems to be particularly useful following cisplatin (Platinol), one of the best-selling cancer drugs. It was only in July of 1982 that the FDA approved Reglan for this sort of use.

A still newer drug that can apparently prevent nausea and vomiting better than any other medication may soon be available in the U.S. The drug, called domperidone, is made by Janssen Pharmaceutica and will be sold under the trade name Motilium. Studies comparing Reglan with Motilium have shown Motilium is more effective. It can cut nausea and vomiting by 96 percent, depending on which anticancer drug is involved in the treatment. Best of all, domperidone appears to have few side effects, even after repeated doses over several weeks.

The active ingredient in marijuana, tetrahydrocannabinol, better known simply as THC, can also prevent the nausea from cancer chemotherapy. Many cancer patients, however, aren't about to start using marijuana to get this relief, and don't care to get high either. A totally synthetic derivative of THC, called nabilone, may overcome these objections. Developed by Eli Lilly, and to be sold under the trade name Cesamet, nabilone has been shown to effectively control nausea with much less euphoria than THC itself. Nabilone is already marketed in Canada and should soon be available in England. It is effective orally and could improve the comfort of many patients undergoing the trauma of cancer chemotherapy.

Food Additives: A Parade of Carcinogens

By now we are quite used to those frequent reports that something we eat has been linked to cancer, mental disorders, birth defects, or some other dreaded problem. It seems that the only safe diet would be bread and water—except that the safety of drinking water has also been questioned.

The number of chemicals in your water will vary, depending on where you live. One of the widespread problems involves chlorination, which is done to kill bacteria and make the drinking water free of disease. But the process of chlorination also produces tiny amounts of chemicals that may cause cancer, and since other purification methods are not yet feasible, it is a problem we are being forced to live with.

Chemicals added to the processed foods we buy, to color them, make them sweeter, preserve them, or for other reasons, have often been found to be cancer causers. Under current law, no chemical that is found to cause cancer in animals—no matter what the dose given to them—can be added to our foods. That is the same law that removed cyclamates, red dye number 2, and DES (diethylstilbesterol) from the market.

The law does not seem to apply all the time, however. Saccharin, for instance, appears to be a weak carcinogen (cancer-causing agent), and under the law should be banned. Yet, political pressure has prevented that step because of the lack of alternatives, although that is now changing.

Another example of the double standard comes out of the nitrite controversy. Nitrites are found naturally in some foods and water and are added to others for flavor and color enhancement, and generally as a preservative. The discovery that cooking meats containing nitrites could cause the formation of nitrosamines (potent cancer causers) started the controversy. Here we had an additive that was not itself a carcinogen but one which might help other carcinogens form. However, removing the nitrites from foods such as bacon and ham could make them susceptible to deadly botulism. The net result seems to be that nitrites will remain in our food but at lower levels.

One of the most recent additives to come under suspicion is blue 2, a chemical dye used mostly in baked goods. Since recent studies have now shown it causes cancer in rats, the odds are that it will be banned—joining several other food colorings in the unemployment line.

A report that diets containing meat might be carcinogenic caused many a vegetarian to gloat and was the source of much anguish in the meat industry. But it appears that vegetarians aren't safe either. One of the most potent carcinogens known is aflatoxin, a natural product from a fungus that can contaminate grain and peanuts. There are legal limits on how much of this substance can remain in our foods, but a zero exposure level is not possible. People on natural diets, where chemicals to kill this fungus are not used and where proper controls are lax, could receive higher levels than desirable.

Through all of this, it is fortunate that the human body has an amazing ability to withstand the chemical onslaught from what we breathe, drink, and eat in twentieth-century life.

Laetrile: R. I. P.

The legend of laetrile now should be laid to rest. Although there was never any evidence of anticancer activity in animals, personal testimonials and public pressure nudged the FDA into conducting tests of laetrile in humans.

Now the human evidence is in and it confirms that laetrile has absolutely no effectiveness in treating cancer. Not only did it turn out to be ineffective against cancer, but it has dangers of its own. Some patients taking it actually showed signs of cyanide poisoning—probably the result of laetrile being degraded to cyanide in the body. Several reports of children dying from cyanide poisoning after eating laetrile confirm the drug's toxicity.

It is tragic that after so many years, cancer victims must still grasp at straws such as laetrile. No one can be blamed for following every avenue, every possibility of a cure. It may be that just such an episode will someday lead to a real breakthrough.

For now, it looks as if we will have to be satisfied with small steps, instead of that one giant leap for mankind.

21

THE CHOLESTEROL CONTROVERSY

Does a diet heavy in cholesterol increase your risk of heart disease? Medical personnel still disagree.

Will drugs that lower your blood cholesterol level help you live longer? There is even more dissension on that point.

Despite the television commercials casting Mr. Cholesterol as the bad guy, and the belief of many scientists that high levels of saturated fat in the blood hasten heart attacks, there is no clear link between dietary fat intake and heart disease.

Even one of the most extensive studies on heart disease risks ever done—a ten-year mammoth effort involving thirteen thousand test subjects—did not answer all the questions. That study, conducted by the National Heart, Lung and Blood Institute, did suggest once again, however, that the risk of heart disease can be reduced by lowering cholesterol levels as well as by reducing blood pressure and quitting smoking.

If there is uncertainty, it is not stopping drug manufacturers. Gemfibrozil, a drug recently approved by the FDA, shows promise as being the first highly effective drug for lowering blood cholesterol. This drug, dubbed Lopid by its manufacturer (Parke-Davis), enters competition with a small number of other cholesterol-lowering agents such as clofibrate (Atromid-S), probucol (Lorelco), and cholestyramine (Questran). All are available by prescription only.

The advantage of gemfibrozil seems to be its ability to raise the level of HDLs (high-density lipoproteins) which is something the other drugs are not able to do. The lipoproteins are a family of molecules that transport cholesterol in the blood. Raising their level can produce high blood cholesterol. The HDLs, as opposed to other lipoproteins, help *reduce* cholesterol deposits while still raising the cholesterol level in the blood.

The ideal treatment of high blood cholesterol would increase HDLs while decreasing the other blood lipoproteins. The preferred way of doing so is by a controlled diet. Only when this fails, as it often does, should drug therapy be used.

Your body does not actually need much additional cholesterol. It produces on its own most of the cholesterol and saturated fat needed for normal growth and development. When dietary intake goes up, the amount manufactured in the body decreases to maintain a balance. Some people's bodies are unable to regulate the amount of fat produced, due to disease or an inherited deficiency. The result can be much higher concentrations of cholesterol and other lipids in the blood, which translates into greater risk of heart attack.

For people with this sort of problem, lowering blood cholesterol levels is a definite plus. There is no doubt that gemfibrozil decreases blood cholesterol and fat. But do not be misled. While high blood cholesterol increases heart attack risk, decreasing the level with drugs for most people does not necessarily lessen the risk. That theory has yet to be proven. The high cholesterol may only be a symptom of something else.

Even with years of research, cholesterol-lowering drugs have not yet proven the theory true, and one study with clofibrate (marketed by Ayerst Laboratories under the trade name Atromid-S) has even suggested an *increased* risk of death because of adverse effects associated with the use of the drug.

A recent study in monkeys has shown that probucol and cholestyramine can stop the atherosclerosis (hardening of the arteries) which normally develops when they eat a diet high in cholesterol. The question remains, however, whether this benefit can be translated to humans eating a normal diet.

One problem doctors face is that simply measuring the cholesterol level is only one item on a list of complex information needed to accurately evaluate the condition of patients whose bodies are unable to control the amount of fat produced.

Lopid (gemfibrozil) is available by prescription because of the importance of monitoring the blood lipid levels and the possible side effects of the drug. Those side effects focus mostly on the gastrointestinal system and include pain, diarrhea, nausea, and vomiting. It is also possible the severe gallbladder problems seen with clofibrate may also appear with gemfibrozil since the two are chemically related. So far that problem has not surfaced and gemfibrozil may indeed be a ground-breaking advance, marking the first truly useful cholesterol-regulating drug.

22

CONTRACEPTIVES: WORKING OUT THE BUGS

The Vindication of the Pill

Birth control pills took a bad rap in recent years but are living on to see their kind vindicated. Not only have a series of studies trickled out which debunk many of the previous fears about health hazards of the pills, but an incredible list of health benefits affecting tens of thousands of women every year has emerged.

Consider some of the claims coming out of a variety of prestigious medical research centers around the world.

- The pill protects women against cancer of the uterus and cancer of the ovaries.
- Pill users are defended against the development of noncancerous breast lumps and cysts.
- Taking the pill can vastly reduce a woman's chances of developing pelvic inflammatory disease (PID).
- The pill affords a degree of protection against a variety of menstrual conditions, including lessening premenstrual pain and tension, and reducing the chances of iron-deficiency anemia.

- Women who are taking the pill have much less of a chance of suffering rheumatoid arthritis.

That is quite a list, and family-planning experts seem to be nothing short of elated about this turnabout in how medical people view birth control pills. This does not even include the fact that birth control pills effectively prevent pregnancy, a highly dangerous condition in itself. It should be quickly pointed out, however, that by no means is the pill free of health risks. But the pendulum has swung in the other direction and the consensus is that the benefits far outweigh the negative aspects.

Estimates place the number of birth control pill users in the United States at about eight million. Since the mid-1970s when the pill scare was running high, many women have turned to alternative methods, fearing the consequences of extended use of birth control pills.

SMOKERS BEWARE

Chief among the risks still associated with use of the pill are heart attacks, blood clots, strokes, high blood pressure, and circulatory diseases. But an overwhelming share of this risk, according to medical reports, falls on women who also smoke. And there is more risk of pill-associated heart disease in women in their mid-forties or older.

The birth control pill is probably one of the most scrutinized drugs in existence. Today's prevailing views about the pill—its diminishing risks and unexpected benefits—are an almost complete reversal of the old fears (not yet erased) about the hazards of using it. What is so remarkable is not only does the pill not seem to cause cancer but it can also offer protection, imperfect though it is, from some types of that dread disease. That is a modern medical miracle of a slightly different bent from what we are used to.

This may be partially attributed to the changes that have been made in the pill, making it safer and more effective. The most dramatic change has been the vast reduction in the amount of the female sex hormones estrogen and progestin (also called progesterone) contained in the pills. The amounts of these hormones are but a fraction of what they were in the early 1970s. This change has not decreased the pill's effectiveness but it has minimized the woman's exposure to these artificial chemicals.

New Contraceptives for Women

The so-called mini-pill is one result of the efforts to cut back on estrogen levels in birth control pills—in this case eliminating estrogen entirely. Women taking mini-pills are taking only a progestin, since estrogen is believed to be responsible for most of the adverse effects associated with the pill. The drawback is their effectiveness in preventing conception, which drops from nearly one hundred percent to about ninety-eight percent. There also seems to be the potential for menstrual problems with this pill since it is taken continually.

Another approach toward dramatically lowering estrogen and progestin levels will be the new high-potency hormones under study, such as norgestimate.

There is also a chance that a controversial drug which has been around since 1967, medroxyprogesterone acetate (Depo-Provera), will become available as a contraceptive. There is no doubt that a single injection of this drug can prevent pregnancy for three months or longer. The problem has been some animal studies suggesting it could cause cancer. However, extensive clinical studies involving more than eleven thousand patients treated for up to eight years have failed to show any increase in cancer.

More than eighty other countries have approved Depo-Provera, seeing it as a reliable, reversible, convenient and, perhaps best of all, long-lasting contraceptive. The fact that a single injection lasts for three months makes it particularly valuable in poor countries and for women who have trouble remembering to take their pill.

It remains questionable whether the FDA will approve this product for use in the United States as a contraceptive, although it is already available as a cancer treatment. The availability of many other effective drugs, and the concern over the safety of Depo-Provera, suggests the answer may be No, in spite of the drug's unique features. Its availability as a cancer drug has spawned a new drug "underground" of women using it as a contraceptive.

Another unique approach that's already being tried in Europe is called the triphasic pill. The idea here is to change the steroid dose taken each day in an attempt to mimic the woman's normal cycle of hormone production. This varied approach results in a lower total steroid dose than is currently available in the lowest fixed-dose contraceptive. This should further reduce the potential for adverse side effects, such as blood clots, hypertension, and altered blood cholesterol levels.

NEW DELIVERY ROUTES

If the drugs themselves are changing, so too are the methods of taking them. It is not just a pill any longer. One extensively studied technique is to implant a capsule beneath the skin which will slowly release the contraceptive. This involves implanting some six capsules, which would prevent fertility for five to six years. However, there may be some loss of effectiveness after the first three or so years.

Happily, since the capsules can be taken out any time, fertility can be restored quickly by removing the drug. What the longer-term impact of such a prolonged hormone treatment would be is still an unknown and there may be other yet undiscovered side effects.

Another convenient delivery route is directly through the vagina. Because the drug is absorbed so well via this route, the dosage can be reduced. Much more of the steroid will reach the ovaries before it is inactivated in the liver, as happens when the pill is taken orally.

The basic product for this is a ring made of a flexible, nonallergenic material called Silastic. The contraceptive steroid is contained in the Silastic, and when the ring is inserted in the vagina, the drug is slowly released. The ring is good for about six months, and there is usually a schedule of three weeks in, one week out, to permit menstruation.

It works very well in preventing pregnancy but like the minipill menstrual problems occur in about eight percent of the women using these rings. Another adverse effect that has been observed is a drop in the level of a substance in the blood that is believed to protect against heart disease produced by cholesterol. There will have to be more research before the rings are approved for use in the United States.

Intrauterine devices (IUDs) are also being retooled to incorporate a contraceptive steroid right in the IUD. The hormone could be released for as long as three years, thus increasing the IUD's effectiveness while decreasing menstrual cramps, bleeding, and infections often seen with standard IUDs.

Only a few of these many developments are available on the market, and some may never get that far. Some of these new products, however, will offer advantages in convenience and effectiveness.

THE CONTRACEPTIVE SPONGE

A new and more effective approach to the use of spermicides is the contraceptive sponge. Sold OTC under the brand name Today for about $1.00 per sponge, as the 2-Day Sponge, it contains a sperm-killing detergent called nonoxynol 9. The sponge is designed to be placed into the vagina and remain there for up to forty-eight hours. It is convenient and seems to be about as effective as the diaphragm.

Because of the length of time this sponge remains in the vagina, there has been some concern about the potential for toxic shock syndrome although nothing has yet been found to support this concern. In fact, there is now some evidence that this sponge can actually prevent some sexually transmitted diseases such as herpes, gonorrhea, and syphilis by killing these along with the sperm.

THE FOUR-TIMES-PER-MONTH PILL

The fast-paced development in the United States of another new discovery, along with similar work being done in Europe, foreshadows a totally new method of birth control. The implications seem enormous for future contraception or as a method of early abortion.

The new drug compounds being tested often do not have names and their components remain closely guarded secrets. But they would have to be taken by a woman only a few days each month, perhaps only four, and could either be taken regularly in the last days of the menstrual cycle or only when pregnancy is suspected—a morning-after pill.

The new four-day pill will work by lowering the level of progesterone in the body when taken for a few days before menstruation. It has the effect of inducing menstruation and preventing pregnancy and is being called a "menstruation regulator" by one manufacturer.

The discovery of a similar compound was first revealed in mid-1982 by a researcher in France. It is a breakthrough that offers a promising new method of regulating the menstrual cycle and controlling human fertility, said French scientist Dr. Etienne-Emile Baulieu in a paper delivered to the French Academy of Sciences.

His compound, known in its early stages as RU-486, is a steroid that acts as an antihormone. Specifically, what it competes against is progesterone, a female sex hormone produced in the ovaries that paves the way in the uterus for development of a fertilized egg. The new compound, as a hormone antagonist, nudges out the progesterone from the uterus. Since progesterone is necessary for pregnancy to occur, none can take place. It was a discovery that confirmed the indispensability of progesterone in maintaining pregnancy.

The likely avenue by which the French discovery will reach the United States is through the American Hoechst Corporation, an affiliate of the French firm which hopes to produce it in Europe.

The French scientist said there is no doubt this new drug can be effective when taken for only a very short period of time. By comparison, the current pill must be taken about three weeks per month or mechanical devices such as an IUD must remain in place permanently.

In the case of confirmed pregnancy, the French compound was also characterized as more effective and psychologically more viable than current methods of abortion. The side effects, although reported to be mild by early research, are still an open question. But it stands to reason that since the steroid pill would be taken only a few days each month, and since the interaction is reversible, the adverse effects can be minimized.

There were some initial failures with the drug among pregnant women in France who volunteered for a test, and researchers explained it as too low a dosage. Actually, dosage, timing, and duration of the new pill are all questions still unanswered. When they are solved, the new four-day pill may live up to the advance billing it is being given by its discoverers.

A Pill for Men: What's the Holdup?

Doesn't it seem strange that scientists have developed all kinds of products women can take that will effectively and reversibly prevent pregnancy, while nothing short of permanent sterilization seems to work for men? Simply put, one of the reasons is that it is far easier to block release of the one egg a woman produces each month than it is to stop the millions of sperm a male body produces daily. A useful product would have to be something that could be taken once a day or less, which would either block sperm production or thwart their ability to move spontaneously, thus preventing fertilization.

At long last some promising advances towards male contraceptives are now showing up. The discovery of gossypol raised considerable hopes for such a product. Gossypol is a chemical accidentally discovered in China when an epidemic of male infertility was traced to uncooked cottonseed oil. Further research turned up gossypol, a natural component of this oil, as the culprit.

That started people thinking that perhaps the substance could be corralled and put to constructive use. There is no doubt as to its effectiveness. After only a few days of treatment the ability of sperm to move is markedly decreased, and after a few weeks the production of sperm also slows down and may stop altogether.

Most of the time things return to normal when gossypol is discontinued. The catch, of course, is the word "most," since in some men the effects may be permanent. That obvious drawback means gossypol itself will never be used commercially. But other related chemicals are being synthesized and one of these may turn out to be superior.

Scientists are not clear on what makes gossypol work the way it does. Some experts think the sperm's ability to move is inhibited by a direct action the chemical exerts on the membrane of the sperm cells. Other evidence from animal studies has shown a decrease in the level of the male hormone testosterone in the blood. This hormone is needed for sperm production. If scientists can make them reversible, drugs that work by either method or both could become the first commercially available and effective male oral contraceptives.

Another route being pursued in this search involves a chemical produced in the brain called luteinizing hormone-releasing hormone, or LHRH. The job of this hormone is to release two other hormones that are needed for normal sperm production. Scientists have discovered that while small amounts of LHRH do the job right, *larger* amounts actually can have the opposite effect—blocking release of the sperm-producing hormones. The problem here is that the male's sex drive is also blunted.

LHRH is also being studied as a contraceptive in women. As in men, large amounts work opposite to what would be expected, and a decrease in fertility occurs. Since LHRH lacks the side effects of regular birth control pills, it may eventually have some use as a contraceptive in women and in men.

A stumbling block: LHRH works best when given daily by injection and it is very expensive. A nasal spray form is currently being tested and it seems to work, although doses one hundred times higher than by injection are needed. Some chemical relatives of LHRH are also being scrutinized for one that will work orally.

In short, do not start looking at the corner drugstore for LHRH or any other male pill anytime soon.

Contraceptive Scoreboard
A Comparison of Effectiveness of Different Contraceptive Methods

Methods	Percentage of Failure Rate	Percentage of Success Rate
Male sterilization	0.02	99.98
Female sterilization	0.13	99.87
Estrogen/progesterone pills:		
Low-dose estrogen	0.27	99.73
High-dose estrogen	0.32	99.68
Progesterone only	1.2	98.8
IUD	1.5	98.5
Diaphragm	1.9	98.1
Condom	3.6	96.4
Coitus interruptus (withdrawal)	6.7	93.3
Spermicides	11.9	88.1
Rhythm method	15.5	84.5

SOURCE: *Lancet,* April 10, 1982.

23

DIABETES CONTROL
SHOWS IMPROVEMENT

The incredibly speedy arrival to the United States of the first human insulin, new methods of taking insulin more accurately, new drugs, and the prospect of cell transplants to cure diabetes are continuing to alter the outlook for treating this disease.

The approval of human insulin is the latest news for diabetics. Until now, insulins have come from either cows or pigs. Those animal insulins can be highly purified but still cause adverse reactions in some diabetics who need to take them.

In 1982, with uncharacteristic lightning quickness, the FDA approved Humulin for use in the United States. Humulin is the Eli Lilly and Company brand name for human insulin that is produced by genetic engineering methods. It was the first genetic engineering success to make it onto the commercial market.

Insulin is a hormone produced in the pancreas. Its function in the body is to help metabolize carbohydrates and fats. A lack of insulin causes the condition we know as diabetes, although doctors now realize diabetes is not caused merely by a lack of insulin.

Insulin that diabetics take to replace what is missing comes in many forms that differ in the speed with which they act and how

148

long they work. This insulin is produced by drug companies from the pancreases of pigs and cows, and the availability of the pig and cow pancreases to make the insulin is tied to demand for meat in the United States. The human insulin that has now arrived may one day totally replace the animal insulins.

Major advances have been made in the animal insulins, however, which could delay the dominance of the human variety. Highly purified preparations are solving the problem of side effects caused by impurities in the animal insulins. Until the mid-1970s, the main contaminant, called proinsulin, could be found at levels over ten thousand parts per million (ppm). Today, the contaminants have been slashed to only about 50 ppm, and can be reduced to less than 10 ppm in highly purified insulins. Elements, such as zinc, added to insulin to improve its ability to function in the body may also be responsible for side effects in some diabetics.

Many diabetics do just fine on the less pure, less expensive animal insulins, and the highly purified preparations are not recommended for everyone. However, about five percent of diabetics who take insulin encounter allergic reactions, showing up as rashes or insulin resistance, forcing larger doses to be taken. The purer insulins and perhaps human insulin can now eliminate much of this problem. Insulin is a natural protein, but some reactions occur because animal insulin differs from human insulin. The difference is slight but it is enough to cause problems for some people.

Gene splicing, known more formally as recombinant DNA technology, provided the way to manufacture human insulin. Basically, it works like this: The genetic information that is responsible for producing insulin in humans is transferred to bacteria. Acting on these new instructions, large vats of these bacteria then function as insulin factories, turning the substance out in large quantities.

Eli Lilly, in conjunction with a West Coast gene-splicing firm called Genentech, has successfully upgraded its production of genetically produced human insulin to commercial levels and other firms are working on doing the same thing. The price, at least in the beginning, will be a little higher than for animal insulins, but the method pretty much assures a bountiful supply in the future— something that was not certain with animal insulins. Diabetics have been advised not to change to human insulin without a doctor's supervision, since a different dose and regimen may be required. Some studies have indicated that human insulin may not remain in the body as long as some of the animal insulins.

In addition to the genetically engineered human insulin, there is another type that will soon join it on the market. This human insulin is made by artificially changing the structure of insulin coming from pigs.

The jury is still out on the advantages of using human insulin. The magazine *Diabetes Forecast* points out that while companies producing human insulin have hoped for a medical advantage to turn up, researchers have not yet proven Humulin to be any better than the very pure animal insulins.

The move toward perfect insulin, which would produce no signs of rejection in the diabetic, remains the goal, although it is one with uncertain prospects.

There is a strong belief that the secret to a cure for diabetes lies in finding a more natural method of administering insulin. Pancreas transplants have brought some success, but also complications because of the other hormones and enzymes produced in this organ. Although still five to ten years away, transplants of pancreatic islet cells (where insulin is produced) seem to offer a better hope for a cure. The transplanted cells would produce insulin as needed, just as in a normal pancreas. Cell transplants of this type have been done successfully in animals.

But they will work differently than other kinds of transplants. Here, islet cells are taken from a pancreas and are injected intravenously into the diabetic subject. Some of the cells will take up residence in the liver, where they function quite nicely. Researchers have also made good progress in solving the inevitable problem of rejection.

NEW WAYS TO TAKE INSULIN

Even with a bountiful supply of pure insulin there is still the problem of how to administer it to avoid wide swings of insulin levels in the blood. It comes down to more of an engineering problem than a medical one.

Tiny insulin pumps that can be implanted in the human body have been developed. In one clinical test, the pump was left in for over nine months without any problems, and with improved control of blood-sugar levels. The test subjects said they preferred the pumps to the otherwise frequent insulin injections. However, these test subjects still had some insulin production ability in their bodies and equal success may not be as easy in people whose bodies make no insulin on their own.

The ultimate implantable pump would continuously monitor blood glucose levels and release insulin as needed, just like a normal pancreas. Devices that do this exist, but they are still far too large to consider implanting.

NEW DIABETES DRUGS

The discovery of insulin in 1921 was heralded as the cure for diabetes. Until that time, diabetics were expected to live only a short time. By giving patients a single large shot of insulin daily to control the blood-sugar level, death has been postponed but not eliminated for the 11 million Americans with this disease. In fact, diabetes remains the third leading death-producing disease.

But the pancreas doesn't release insulin in a big lump. The large swings in insulin levels caused by such injections are partly to blame for the most serious complications in diabetics including blindness, blood-vessel disease, and kidney failure.

There has been great improvement in recent years, but diabetic complications still occur.

A new oral drug in the final stages of clinical testing, sorbinil, from Pfizer Pharmaceuticals, has shown the ability to prevent or even reverse some of the severe complications of diabetes. It has no effect on diabetes itself, but can prevent the eye damage and possible blindness caused by diabetes. It can also prevent damage to the kidney, blood vessels and heart. If sorbinil is proven safe and effective, diabetics may soon be taking it along with insulin.

Other new drugs include a second generation of chemicals which lower blood sugar (oral hypoglycemics). These drugs seem to help the body metabolize glucose directly and stimulate the release of insulin. They are helpful only in less severe forms of diabetes where the pancreas can still make some insulin. They don't provide a cure, nor do these drugs prevent long term complications. Combined with a strict diet, however, they can allow some diabetics to eliminate the insulin shots.

Five such drugs are currently marketed in Europe. Several under study for possible approval in the United States include glipizide, which would be marketed by Pfizer as Glucotrol, and gliburide, which Upjohn would sell as Macronase and which would also be marketed by the American Hoechst Corporation.

24

DIARRHEA: BEST ADVICE MAY NOT BE DRUGS

Former President Jimmy Carter probably did more to publicize traveler's diarrhea than anyone else with his infamous Montezuma's Revenge remark, made while he was visiting Mexico. It is called *turista,* or the trots, but by whatever name, it has ruined more vacations than lost travelers checks.

Traveler's diarrhea is usually caused by local micro-organisms that invade your gastrointestinal tract. Of course, lots of bacteria normally live in your intestines, but the foreign invaders upset the delicate balance of events, resulting in up to eight watery bowel movements every day. Preventing diarrhea becomes a passion with some American travelers. Concern and care are warranted, but the odds are actually even or slightly in your favor, as only twenty-five to fifty percent of North American visitors to Mexico develop diarrhea.

What can you do if you are among those who do not beat the odds? Antibiotics are sometimes recommended as more evidence points to their effectiveness in preventing or curing traveler's diarrhea. However, some diarrhea is caused by viruses or parasites that will not respond to the antibiotics and it usually goes away in a few days anyway. There is also fear that the widespread use of antibiotics for prevention will enhance the development of bacteria resistant to these drugs, making treatment of more severe cases difficult.

Nevertheless, new evidence suggests that taking a combination of two antibiotics, trimethoprim and sulfamethoxazole (this combination is available under the brand names Bactrim and Septra) may prevent or cure attacks of this uncomfortable problem.

Still, antibiotics only work against certain types of bacteria and if your diarrhea is not caused by the type of bacteria the antibiotic you are taking can kill, you are out of luck. Side effects are another strike against antibiotics for diarrhea. They are potent drugs and people sensitive or allergic to them can develop severe reactions. This is true not only with trimethoprim-sulfamethoxazole, but also with ampicillin and doxycycline (Pfizer's Vibramycin, the most popular brand name), both of which have been used against traveler's diarrhea and seem to be effective.

With ampicillin and doxycycline in particular, there has been concern that they will kill off the good bacteria in the intestine, thus making it even easier for the bad ones to take over. In other words, the antibiotics might give initial relief but actually make things worse later on.

With doxycycline it is also possible to permanently stain the teeth of children and it should not be taken by kids under seven years of age or by pregnant women. If your plans include getting lots of exposure to sunlight, you will also have to be careful if using doxycycline. Severe skin reactions due to increased sun sensitivity are common, especially for travelers to tropical countries.

Once diarrhea begins, many travelers try to treat it with preparations such as Lomotil, which slows the movement of the intestinal tract, or a bulk-forming agent such as Metamucil, which tends to make the stools less liquid. Travelers report some relief, but many doctors believe these drugs will also prolong the overall effects of the diarrhea and that they should be used sparingly and cautiously.

Perhaps the most important thing to remember is to take in plenty of fluids to offset the considerable loss from the diarrhea. A relatively mild case of diarrhea can quickly become a severe case of dehydration if this step is not followed.

Far and away the best advice is to prevent the diarrhea in the first place. That is not always possible, but watching what you eat helps.

In foreign countries, beware of anti-diarrhea drug products sold locally. Some products available elsewhere are harmful and have been banned in the United States while others are very potent and should only be used under a physician's supervision. Remember also that quality control in other countries may not be as effective as in the United States.

The best way to avoid an attack of diarrhea is to eat only cooked foods and fresh fruits that can be peeled. Other fresh fruits and vegetables will have been washed in the local water, which is usually the source of the offending organisms. Drink only bottled beverages and avoid ice cubes—they are made using local water. Most attacks begin three to five days after a visitor arrives and last anywhere from one to four days, although some people never seem to shake the problem. Accompanying gas pains, cramps, nausea, fever, and headaches can make it an uncomfortable experience.

25

DIET AIDS: YOU CAN'T FOOL MOTHER NATURE

The Cruel Myth of Diet Aids

Taking drugs or so-called diet aids to help lose weight has become a routine practice in the United States. The cruel myth that diet drugs can help is perpetuated by the manufacturers and sellers of a large variety of dieting products, while studies of weight loss prove otherwise.

Scientists can create new life forms and perform medical miracles on the human body, but beyond the simple explanation that we get fat by absorbing more calories than we burn up, modern medicine is at a loss to help in weight loss.

Trying to lose weight can be frustrating. There just aren't any easy ways to reverse the biological process by which our bodies gain extra poundage. Losing weight has always and still does require severe mental and physical discipline. Millions of people wanting to shed pounds have sought help through pharmaceutical crutches, otherwise known as diet aids. Private enterprise keeps coming to the rescue with its extensive menu of these big-selling,

OTC products designed to help people lose weight by curbing the appetite. Unfortunately, the procedure is not nearly as simple as taking a few appetite suppressants and, presto, the pounds begin to drop off.

If your goal is long-term weight loss (getting it off and keeping it off) as well as good health, at best the OTC diet aids available could prove to be only marginally helpful in curbing your appetite, and even then for only a few weeks. At worst, the drugs you take can be harmful.

Any hope of losing weight would have to include some kind of planned diet in addition to the drugs. Yet Americans keep spending millions of dollars every year on weight-loss promoters. The most basic misconception is that the diet aids make you lose pounds. They do not. They are simply supposed to help you eat less, although just how effective they are in that regard has been questioned.

HOW THE PROCESS WORKS

Scientists have tried to figure out how hunger, and its opposite in the body, satiety, work. Research findings suggest that there are two separate centers of the brain that control eating. One tells us when and how much to eat. The other signals when to stop.

One theory claims that your weight is controlled by the balance between these two centers. That would make your body essentially preprogrammed to a particular level of fatness. In fact, just which level you come out on might be hereditary.

Plugging in a new program can be difficult if not impossible in the long run. Your body is content to stay the way it is. When you try to diet, it may fight back by trying to follow the original blueprint it was given. You end up trying to fool your own system into becoming thinner. Initial success in outfoxing your system might come easy but deceptively so. Getting your body to stay in line over a long period of time is what can be so tough.

The drugs sold as OTC diet aids simply cannot keep on fooling your system for very long. Your body catches on within a few weeks and begins to ignore the chemical instructions delivered by the drugs.

The only effective and permanent way to shed excess weight would be to change your body's idea of what it should weigh. That is essentially where medical science fails us. Although no such means to alter the blueprint has been found, sustained exercise seems to come closest.

Amphetamines, which are now strictly controlled by the government, were once the most widely used appetite-control drugs. Amphetamines fall into a class known as sympathomimetics and their target is the appetite center, located in the lower region of the brain known as the hypothalamus. One of their major drawbacks is that the ability to decrease your appetite only lasts two or three weeks. Exactly why this happens is not known, but scientists believe the brain adapts to the intrusion of the foreign substance and goes back to functioning the way it did before the drug arrived.

Since you are merely stimulating nerves artificially by taking the drug, the body adjusts. The process is similar to the stimulation of your smell nerves. When you are in a room with a strong odor you stop noticing it after a few hours because the body adapts to the stimulation. The difference with diet aids is that the adjustment takes a bit longer.

If you were to stop taking the drug for several weeks, the appetite suppressant effect would return. But such on-and-off dieting usually results in regaining any weight that was lost.

The reputation of amphetamines as uppers, or pep pills, is not without foundation either. Once they reach the brain, they unlock a chemical called norepinephrine that is stored naturally in your nerve terminals. It is this chemical, released by natural processes, that is responsible for transmitting nerve impulses through the body.

Amphetamines stimulate the part of the brain that elevates mood and also suppresses the appetite center. The trouble is this euphoria often results in a severe psychological dependence on the drug.

Because of this, the FDA keeps a tight lid on the sale and use of amphetamines. They are classified as a Schedule Two drug, meaning a written prescription is necessary and no refills are permitted without a new prescription.

SIMILAR OTC DRUG WIDELY USED

The abuse potential of amphetamines has pushed them to the back shelf for appetite control, but a close cousin—both chemically and in the way it works—is widely available without a prescription in a variety of diet aids. This drug, phenylpropanolamine (PPA), works by prolonging the nerve-stimulating effects of norepinephrine (the neurotransmitter already in your body). Like amphetamines, phenylpropanolamine can also stimulate the release of extra amounts of that chemical in the body.

Some of the common OTC products containing phenylpropanolamine include: Anorexin, Appredrin, Ayd's AM/PM, Cenadex, Control, Dexatrim, Diadax, Dietac, and Spantrol.

Since this drug's ability to actually stimulate activity in the brain is limited, so too is its potential for abuse. It is more difficult to become psychologically addicted to phenylpropanolamine and that is one reason it is available without a prescription. It will suppress the appetite center, but with continuous use the effect wears off in just two to three weeks. For long-term weight control, its usefulness is questionable.

Why then has the FDA classified this drug as safe and effective, a designation few drugs have achieved? Because the FDA requires only two things: that the drug is safe (which it probably is) and that it does what the manufacturer says it does. Contrary to popular belief, the FDA is not concerned with whether the drug will actually cause you to lose weight or whether the appetite-dampening effect lasts beyond three weeks.

Interestingly, phenylpropanolamine is also used as a nasal decongestant because it constricts blood vessels, which in turn decreases swelling and mucus secretion.

The problems with this drug get serious when too much is taken. Some dieters seem to think that if one works well, two or three will work even better. The resulting excess stimulation of the central nervous system can show up as nervousness, insomnia, or nausea. The constriction of blood vessels can increase blood pressure, which is especially dangerous since high blood pressure is already common among overweight individuals.

Phenylpropanolamine, an ingredient you can find in over seventy varieties of nasal decongestants and diet pills, has also been linked to severe kidney problems and muscle damage. One report appearing in the *Journal of the American Medical Association* suggested that use of the drug should be completely reconsidered. Other medical organizations have suggested that phenylpropanolamine be made a prescription drug because of the purported health threats.

Manufacturers have disputed the claimed adverse effects on blood pressure and continue to maintain that diet aids containing phenylpropanolamine are contributing to weight loss in people using them.

THE MYSTERIES OF FAT

At the biochemical level, defining the process of getting fat is deceivingly simple: the body absorbs more calories than it burns up. Of course, two people eating exactly the same food and burning up exactly the same number of calories might not maintain the same weight. Some bodies use food more efficiently than others, which is why one person seems to gain a pound with each slice of bread while another does not gain an ounce on three hamburgers and a milkshake.

The standard rule is that you must absorb thirty-five hundred excess calories to gain one pound of fat. From the other angle, it means you must eat at least five hundred fewer calories each day than you burn up to lose one pound in a week. But even counting calories is deceiving. Your body wants to keep that fat, and faced with a shortage it might start hanging on to more of what it is offered.

Within the next few years, dieters may also be seeing new synthetic fat-substitute products appearing on the market—the fruits of experimental research now ongoing. One such product, sucrose polyester, is not absorbed at all by the body when consumed and therefore has absolutely no calories. Whether it is a food additive or a weight-loss aid, it will need FDA approval, probably as a drug and probably by prescription. No doubt it will also be given a more appealing name by the time it reaches the commercial market.

Procter & Gamble holds the patent on this substance that can be used in place of cooking oils or milk fat. Once again this substance is supposed to fool the body by passing right on through without being absorbed. Its unique synthetic molecular structure is supposed to accomplish that trick. Preliminary studies in overweight patients have shown that while they eat the same amount, what they consume has 500 fewer calories, so they lose weight.

A more exotic way to help people lose weight is being pursued by three major drug firms—Eli Lilly, Burroughs Wellcome, and Hoffmann-LaRoche. These companies are looking for a drug which will mimic the effects of exercise, forcing the body to burn off excess fat. The process is known as thermogenesis, since a slight fever is produced by effective drugs.

Previous efforts in this area resulted in effective but highly toxic drugs. The aim now is to get rid of these dangerous side effects, although many researchers believe it cannot be done.

As scientists learn more about how appetite is controlled in the brain, drug companies are rushing to use this knowledge to come up with new and more effective drugs to chemically suppress your desire to eat.

OTHER AIDS AND INGREDIENTS

Nerve stimulators are not the only drugs promoted as diet aids. The bulk-forming agents, such as methylcellulose and carboxymethylcellulose, bloat up in the stomach to produce a full feeling. They are safe since nothing is absorbed into the body. But the amount used is normally far too small to do any good, and it disappears from the stomach within thirty minutes and can sometimes act like a laxative. The latest fad product in this area that became a big seller is glucomannan, a pill made of fibers extracted from a sort of root.

One rather bizarre ingredient that has been used in some OTC diet aids is benzocaine, a local anesthetic. It is the same stuff you put on your skin to stop sunburn pain, in the form of Solarcaine or other similar products. In chewable diet aids the idea is to numb your mouth, alter your normal tastes, and thus lessen your appetite. In capsules or tablets, it is supposed to deaden your stomach in order to suppress the appetite. However, there is no evidence that benzocaine has any effect on your appetite in any way.

Most diet aids, especially the ones containing phenylpropanolamine, contain other ingredients, including liberal amounts of caffeine and sometimes vitamins. The amount of caffeine varies, but usually equals what you'd get in one or two cups of coffee.

The caffeine is there not for any appetite-inhibiting effects, but merely for the stimulation of the nervous system. The caffeine lift works differently than the one you get from the other drug, but the result is the same, mood elevation, which can be enhanced by the phenylpropanolamine. That can lead to both physical and psychological dependence, just as many people need that first cup of coffee in the morning to get going.

Some individuals actually experience withdrawal symptoms from their caffeine dependence which manifests itself in severe head-aches. This could happen with the diet aids containing caffeine, especially if you are getting caffeine from other sources such as coffee, tea, and soft drinks. Caffeine is also suspected of aggravating the symptoms of fibrocystic breast disease, which is common among young women. (For more details see Chapter 19, *Caffeine or No Caffeine?*)

The more natural way to lose weight will require changing your eating and exercise lifestyle and keeping it up. The drugs cannot help unless accompanied by that discipline, so why use them? The natural way is undoubtedly healthier and more effective than phar-maceutical crutches.

Starch Blockers: Too Good to be True (and not)

There is a very powerful sales lure behind any drug that would help you lose weight and at the same time let you eat as much or even more than usual of your favorite foods. Such a highly sought-after product would substitute chemistry for willpower and exer-cise and allow individuals to overeat without guilt.

Claims that just such a miracle product exists abounded with the sudden introduction of starch blockers. People in the market for diet aids may have come across some of the more than three dozen brands of starch blockers that blanketed the market (before they were banned), being sold under such names as Red-U-Cal, Blok-Cal, Starch Breaker, Calorex, Starch Block, and Sta-Trim. Health food and drugstore windows started featuring signs offering miracle diet products that would eliminate the dieter's nightmare of starchy foods. Bookstores quickly stocked up on the books on starch blocker diets. Advertisements for mail-order pills abounded.

The government's watchdog agency in such matters, the FDA, took a dim view and in mid-1982 moved to ban the sale of starch-blocker products until more could be learned about their safety. Long after the FDA's action, however, some manufacturers were not complying, pending legal challenges, and starch blockers remained on store shelves and the books remained in the bookstores.

Finally, a federal court banned the manufacture and sale of starch blockers and the government seized inventories of the drug. But the starch blockers could be back as various appeals work their way through our judicial system.

The starch blockers became a fad product with dieters and, as with other fad items, were made without government control, raising the possibility of impurities. They are made from raw kidney and northern beans, which contain some toxic chemicals (and possibly other ingredients as yet unknown, even to the FDA). These poisons could cause problems for people taking improperly processed starch blockers.

The theory behind how starch blockers are supposed to work goes like this: A protein which can inhibit the action of the digestive enzyme amylase is extracted from the beans and made into the starch-blocker pill. In the body, amylase normally breaks down starch into glucose so it can be absorbed. Without that action by the enzyme, the starch would pass right through the intestine without ever providing the body with any usable calories.

The theory may be simple, but putting it into practice is not. A recent study in *The New England Journal of Medicine* failed to find any change in the number of calories absorbed by people taking these products. There are several possible explanations for this. Since this starch blocker is really a protein, it will be digested along with the other proteins you eat—probably before it has much of a chance to work as a starch blocker. Even under ideal conditions in the laboratory, each tablet can only eliminate about four hundred calories of starch. Any significant or prolonged weight loss would still require some sort of dietary control.

Some products sold as starch blockers contained virtually none of the desired starch-blocking protein and consumers ended up paying high prices for little more than powdered kidney beans.

Another caution comes from nutritionists. They say that if starch consumption is blocked, the calories needed by the body will have to come from somewhere else, namely fat and protein. But exclusive metabolism of those foods for energy could be dangerous. Diabetics would face a grave danger as they would be unable to accurately calculate the number of usable calories they are consuming while taking starch blockers.

The companies that were making and selling starch blockers had bypassed the FDA by calling the product a food supplement instead of a drug. The normal process required to test a drug for effectiveness and safety is, of course, very time-consuming and expensive. The issue was actually quite clear cut, however, since federal law classifies a substance as a drug if it is offered for non-food purposes and it alters a function of the body. A federal judge later said that simply because the product is derived from a natural food does not preclude government regulation of it as a drug.

One reason the government stepped in was the increasing level of consumer complaints involving starch blockers. Those complaints included nausea, vomiting, diarrhea, and gas pains. Interestingly, however, these are precisely the effects that would suggest the starch blockers are working as claimed. The problem is this: Once the undigested starch reaches the large intestine, bacteria present there will begin to eat it, thus producing the adverse effects people are complaining of.

The field of diet medicine is full of remedies aimed at the large numbers of people who put themselves through desperate and recurring efforts to lose weight. It seems likely the starch blockers' promise of easy weight loss really was too good to be true. Weight control is a complex problem that may never have an easy answer.

In spite of all the hype, the best way to lose weight is still a well-planned diet under a physician's supervision combined with a highly motivated individual.

Aspartame: How Sweet it is

Combine two amino acids in the laboratory in just the right way and what do you get? The answer is aspartame, the new artificial sweetener that is 180 times sweeter than sugar and has now been approved for use in the United States.

Aspartame is especially good news for dieters or people who must stay away from sugar for other medical reasons. The impetus for finally bringing it on the market came in 1977 when some researchers in Canada announced that long-term use of high doses of saccharin might lead to cancer.

The uproar that followed was understandable since saccharin was still the only artificial sweetener available in this country. Suddenly, the FDA banned saccharin and tried to make it a behind-the-counter drugstore item, carrying the label of a suspected cause of cancer. Without anything to fill the void, Congress stepped in to prevent that ban from going into effect—a move that remains in force today.

It now looks like aspartame will be used extensively as a safe sugar substitute in items ranging from chewing gum to breakfast cereals, and as a tablet or powder on the dinner table.

Aspartame was much slower in finding its way into diet soft drinks in the United States, but that use has now gained FDA approval as well. According to reports from Canada, where aspartame has been used to sweeten diet soft drinks since 1981, that should be a welcome change for dieters' taste buds. Consumers are having a difficult time telling the difference between aspartame and real sugar, and they say there's no comparison with the poorer taste of saccharin. Consumption of diet sodas in Canada soared after the introduction of aspartame.

One big roadblock was cost. Aspartame costs nearly twenty times more than saccharin, so American soft-drink manufacturers are leery of spending the extra money. A possible course will be for the soft-drink makers to use a combination of saccharin and aspartame to keep the cost down yet improve the taste.

The other key problem is the length of time aspartame remains stable when it is in liquid form for about six months. What happens then? The aspartame starts to lose its sweetness, which could lead to some very surprised consumers. Manufacturers are loath to have their drinks spoil on the shelf.

The powdered, or table-top form of aspartame is now being marketed as Equal by G. D. Searle and Company, a large drug firm. The bulk product is known as NutraSweet. Although aspartame itself is not entirely free of calories, it is so sweet that only tiny amounts need to be used to obtain the desired sweetness. One calorie of aspartame will replace about 160 calories worth of regular sugar.

Aspartame is actually an artificial combination of two amino acids: aspartic acid and phenylalanine. Saccharin, on the other hand, is a synthetic chemical created in the lab. Amino acids are natural chemicals that form the building blocks of the proteins found in all animals.

Although aspartame itself is technically an artificial product, its components have natural origins and this suggests it will be safe to use. The research on aspartame has supported this assumption, but there is at least one group that should avoid using it. These are the people who suffer the rare genetic disorder phenylketonuria. This disease prevents the body from breaking down phenylalanine, which is one of the amino acids used to make aspartame.

Aspartame was first discovered in 1965 and the extremely long delay in getting it approved for use in the United States was at least partly the result of one early study that suggested massive doses might increase the chance of brain tumors. Fortunately, many studies done since that time were unable to verify that claim and aspartame should be quite a useful sugar substitute. But it may not be the only alternative for long.

Remember the big uproar over cyclamates, the artificial sweeteners that were suspected of causing cancer and were banned by the FDA back in 1973? Well, the drug firm Abbott Laboratories, which made cyclamates, keeps trying to bring them back. Abbott's latest effort claims new evidence that cyclamates can be used safely. Over forty countries currently allow the substance on the market and there seems to be a chance the FDA will reapprove them.

The latest idea to regain approval in the United States is to combine cyclamates with other noncaloric sweeteners to dilute any possible harmful effects. Such combinations were in fact used before cyclamates were banned. The combination makes the resulting product much sweeter as well, so even lesser amounts need be used. Abbott says it would limit the risk of your being poisoned by any one of the food additives, which might also again include saccharin. Keep an eye out for this one as well as another sweetener under development called acesulfame K.

26

FIGHTING THE
UNGLAMOROUS FUNGUS

Among the most unpleasant, not to mention the most difficult human infections to cure, is the lowly fungus. Just about everybody is familiar with the common fungal infections such as athlete's foot and jock itch (caused by a ringworm fungus). But there are plenty of other varieties including the rare and sometimes fatal fungal infections called blastomycosis, histoplasmosis, coccidioidomycosis, and cryptococcosis. They can attack people whose natural defenses have been damaged or suppressed by drugs.

A fungus, whether it carries one of these exotic names or not, is a disease that invades the human body, grows, and can cause some bizarre and disfiguring infections. Effective drugs to fight them have been distressingly slow in appearing on the pharmaceutical market. One reason is that fungal cells are similar in many ways to normal human cells. Designing and building a drug that will recognize the fungus and attack it but not harm other normal cells that look similar has presented problems.

There are a few useful drugs, including one new, highly effective antifungal agent called ketoconazole. Aside from the fact that it works well, the main advantage that ketoconazole has over earlier drugs is that it can be taken orally.

Having an antifungal drug in oral form now eliminates some of the practical problems of trying to fight a fungal infection with long-term drug therapy. Like many of the older drugs, ketoconazole must be given for months or even years to do its job right. But unlike some of those older products which had to be given intravenously, this drug will work orally.

The trade name for this product is Nizoral, made by Janssen Pharmaceutica, a subsidiary of Johnson & Johnson. It works by preventing the fungus cell from producing ergosterol, which is the fungus' answer to cholesterol. Without this fat, the fungus cells start to leak, and become weak enough for the human body's natural defenses to finish off the task of destroying them.

However, ketoconazole will only be absorbed into the system from the stomach if there is enough stomach acid present. That means you should not take this drug at the same time you are taking antacids or ulcer medications such as Tagamet. Those other medications will decrease the amount of stomach acid present, thus preventing the antifungus drug from being absorbed into the system. The result, of course, is that it would not work. If taken correctly, ketoconazole works against many kinds of fungus but not all of them. Unfortunately, the ones it fails to affect are some of the worst ones.

A bonus benefit that this drug offers is that fungal cells do not become resistant to it. On the negative side, however, some patients suffer relapses once the treatment is stopped.

Ketoconazole has not been approved for treating fungal infections of the skin, such as ringworm, but it seems very effective against them. In fact, treating fungal infections of the skin may ultimately become ketoconazole's major use, especially the fungi that have become resistant to the older drugs currently in use such as griseofulvin.

Ketoconazole has another advantage in having fewer side effects than the older antifungal drugs. Nausea, vomiting, and appetite loss are the most frequent side effects, affecting up to twenty percent of the people taking the drug. Liver damage is the most serious potential danger, but it is very rare, occurring only .01 percent of the time.

Other new antifungal drugs being developed should also provide some relief. Tioconazole, sold by Pfizer Laboratories as Trosyd, and butaconozole and sulconazole to be sold by Syntex Laboratories, should be effective topical and vaginal antifungal drugs. Also of interest is bifonazole which is presently being tested and is promising against several fungal diseases.

Ketoconazole and these other drugs certainly are not among the glamor drugs receiving all the attention, but they are a significant improvement for treating a fungal disease. They offer the prospect of a more pleasant cure for these unpleasant infections.

27

GALLSTONES:
A NEW DRUG
INSTEAD OF SURGERY?

New drugs sometimes do not live up to their initial billing, and one such case involves the search for a drug that can dissolve gallstones. Such a product could eliminate the need for many gall-stone operations—one of the leading surgical procedures performed in the United States. This is a story that can be looked at both as a disappointment and as a hopeful beginning toward finding an effective gallstone-dissolving drug.

The main character is chenodeoxycholic acid, also known as chenodiol or CDCA. When it was first discovered that chenodiol appeared favorable in dissolving gallstones, it was offered up as the drug that could finally eliminate virtually all need for gallstone operations. That was a gross overestimation. When the extensive study results recently started coming in, it turned out that chenodiol is not nearly as effective as was promised early on.

That was a major disappointment for some fifteen million Americans who suffer from gallstones. Millions more are said to have them and not know it. These are known as silent stones.

It has been estimated that one million new gallstone cases will be diagnosed this year, and that hundreds of thousands of people will have their gallbladders surgically removed. In spite of test results that didn't live up to expectations, FDA approval for the introduction of this drug in the United States was expected.

The gallbladder acts as a container for the collection of bile produced in the liver, and while the gallbladder is important to digestion, your body is able to get along without it if it is surgically removed. The stones can develop when bile production is abnormal, or when there is an infection in the gallbladder. This in turn can cause chemicals in the bile—particularly cholesterol—to crystallize. About eighty percent of all gallstones are cholesterol gallstones, and this is the variety that the drug chenodiol is supposed to be able to dissolve. The stones can vary in size—from pinpoint size to the size of a grape—and can be present in numbers up to a hundred. The chances of developing gallstones increase with age, and women are three to four times more likely to develop gallstones than men.

The initial encouraging reports on chenodiol said that up to fifty percent of gallstone sufferers taking the drug would have their stones completely dissolved. The big blow came with the results of a much larger two-year study, the National Cooperative Gallstone Study, that was recently completed. That study brought the cure rate for chenodiol down sharply. It now looks like the drug can totally dissolve gallstones only about fourteen percent of the time. About sixty percent of patients given the drug experience no change at all. What is worse, the substance was found to increase blood cholesterol levels, which could increase the risk of heart disease.

A debate over the drug was touched off. According to the manufacturer, Rowell Laboratories, Inc., located in Minnesota, newer follow-up studies are showing better results. Critics of the National Cooperative Gallstone Study, which greatly lowered expectations for the drug, say the dosage levels used were far too low to do any good. They point out that small stones were dissolved best, while the larger ones proved resistant to the low dosage of the drug. Published reports on the drug indicate that the size of the gallstone has a great deal to do with how long the drug must be taken, and whether or not it will work.

The silver lining in this otherwise disappointing scenario is that some patients *were* cured, proving that drug treatment can be used to dissolve gallstones. It seems logical that this substance should prove useful in some way, since chenodiol is one of three acids that exist naturally in the human bile. Patients are required to take the drug for anywhere from six months to several years to get results.

Apparently, it was the positive side of the affair that led an FDA advisory committee to unanimously recommend approval of chenodiol for use in the United States, joining more than forty other countries where the drug is in use. Rowell Laboratories will market the drug under the trade name Chenix.

People who take the drug should be aware that while it is a natural product, the high doses that are likely to be used are not without side effects. Diarrhea is one of those side effects, and strikes about four in every ten people taking the drug. Liver damage also seems to occur in some individuals.

The main benefits of chenodiol seem to be in people who cannot or will not undergo surgery. If symptoms continue in spite of drug treatment, surgery is necessary. But that does not mean that everyone who discovers they have gallstones needs surgery. A mere eighteen percent of people with gallstones ever have any problems, which probably means surgery is only needed if symptoms appear. Many of the gallstone operations being performed in the United States are unnecessary.

Even as enthusiasm for chenodiol somewhat wanes, a related drug is receiving more attention. Ursodeoxycholic acid, or ursodiol, seems to be more potent than chenodiol, and perhaps more effective. Better yet, ursodiol causes much less diarrhea and liver damage.

One question that has yet to be answered about either of these gallstone-dissolving drugs is whether the cures achieved are permanent. Some recent work suggests the answer is no, as about half of the "cured" patients will again develop gallstones. Fortunately, these new gallstones can often be dissolved with a new course of drug treatment.

It seems likely that additional research will turn up new, safer, and more effective gallstone-dissolving drugs. In the meantime, chenodiol is a beginning and ursodiol a promising second step to avoid surgery for gallstones.

28

HEART AND BLOOD DRUGS: A REVOLUTION COMES OF AGE

Tracking the Nation's Number-One Killer

In 1940, the leading cause of death in the United States was heart disease. That didn't change in 1960, 1970, or 1980. Today, heart disease is still responsible for over half of all deaths in the United States.

Something good is happening, however. Deaths due to heart disease are dropping, and the pace of that decline in recent years has accelerated. There are many reasons for this turnaround, not the least of which is, simply, an awareness of the problem. One of the most important reasons is the onslaught of many new drugs that have not only helped add years to the average lifespan, but have improved the quality of those added years as well. The United States is a world leader in this area. Other countries have not matched American strides against heart disease, taken in a variety of directions.

Many of the latest pharmaceutical developments in the fight to reduce the toll taken by heart and blood disorders are covered in this chapter. They include entirely new categories of drugs that have revolutionized the treatment of heart disease and high blood pressure (hypertension); new oral drugs as well as the new through-the-skin delivery system of nitroglycerin that can *prevent* angina attacks rather than just stop them once they've started; and single drugs now available for use against several different kinds of heart disease.

There are some as yet unclassified new products—the first real advances in two hundred years—to treat congestive heart failure, the most common of heart diseases. There are surprising new blood clot liquefiers which, when used in radical new ways, can stop heart attacks *in progress,* potentially saving many lives. There are new choices of drugs to control high blood pressure, for people who do not respond well or experience intolerable side effects from other drugs. Even some old drugs are finding new uses against a variety of cardiovascular diseases.

In the midst of it all, there are also major new concerns about side effects of some of the heart drugs, controversies over unwarranted claims, and some surprising new study findings about cutting heart disease risks.

Viewed together, these developments represent a vastly changed and still rapidly advancing field of medicine that affects tens of millions of Americans. There is still room for improvement, but in more and more cases, heart disease is a problem that can be understood and controlled.

Angina: Calcium Channel Blockers to the Rescue

There is a new family of heart drugs on the market that television and movie producers are not going to like. They are known as the calcium channel blockers and they include the first three oral forms of a highly effective medicine for treating angina—the sensation of a life-threatening, crushing pain in the chest.

The newly marketed drugs threaten to make obsolete one of the dramatic staples of the film industry: the sudden collapse of a main character who, suffering an angina attack, gropes desperately for a bottle of nitroglycerin pills. After some tense moments, the attack subsides.

Nitroglycerin is rapidly absorbed by the body when placed under the tongue and will quickly stop an anginal seizure by expanding arteries and increasing blood flow. Nitroglycerin taken this way is not effective in *preventing* such attacks in the first place, however. That is where the calcium blockers come in. When the three oral products which can effectively prevent anginal attacks received government approval recently, they may have taken away the film-maker's dramatic tool.

The movie-makers got away with this ploy longer than they should have anyway. Belated government approval for use of these drugs in the United States seems a classic case of drug lag, resulting from the FDA's lengthy procedures for approving new drugs. The calcium blockers—diltiazem, sold by Marion Laboratories as Cardizem, nifedipine, marketed by Pfizer Inc. under the trade name Procardia, and verapamil, sold by Searle Pharmaceuticals Inc. as Calan and by Knoll Pharmaceutical Co. as Isoptin—have been used successfully in Europe for nearly two decades. Patients and clinicians here have long awaited their arrival to this side of the Atlantic.

The key to drug treatment of angina is its cause, a temporary lack of oxygen reaching the heart due to a narrowing of the blood vessels (hardening of the arteries) and spasms of these same vessels. Angina symptoms only appear when all of the heart's normal reserve capacity has been taken up.

By this time, however, even mild exertion from exercise, cold weather, emotional stress, or even overeating can induce an oxygen imbalance in the heart. The ensuing anginal seizure normally lasts only a few minutes, but the severe pain and unpredictability have prompted a search for better drug treatments.

Nitroglycerin, along with the drug propranolol in more recent years, have carried the burden of treating angina pectoris. They are highly effective but unable to help some patients.

Nifedipine, diltiazem, and verapamil attack the problem from a different angle; they are effective in *preventing* anginal attacks in most patients, including those resistant to other kinds of therapy. Taken orally, these drugs stop the arterial spasms causing the pain by partially blocking the flow of calcium ions in the heart—hence the term calcium blockers. There are calcium channels in the membranes of cells and the calcium is needed for the muscle cells to contract. Block the flow of calcium and you prevent contractions or seizures.

A group of drugs that has been around longer and is used to prevent angina attacks is the beta blocker family. Some members treat angina while others are used for high blood pressure. They work by slowing down the heart or cutting back on its appetite for oxygen. (See the sections that follow, "The Magic of Beta Blockers" and "Differences Among Beta Blockers," for a description of new developments here.)

Another consideration, according to the manufacturer's information on the beta blockers is this: people recently taken off of them might develop a withdrawal syndrome with a resulting increase in angina. Pfizer points out that using Procardia will not prevent this, and could actually make it worse. They suggest a more gradual withdrawal from beta blockers before starting to use a drug such as Procardia.

However, according to Pfizer, when used against one particular type of angina, Procardia eliminated attacks altogether in sixty-three percent of the patients. Another twenty-four percent of patients had their attacks reduced by more than half.

CONTROVERSY ERUPTS

It was not long after Pfizer got its promotional efforts for Procardia in full swing that the company was accused by the FDA of false and misleading advertising of the drug. Among other things, Pfizer had been claiming that Procardia was better than verapamil (Calan and Isoptin), and that it could be taken safely with beta blockers. The FDA challenged the assertion that Procardia can be effective against angina when other drugs fail. The FDA also points out that there are potentially dangerous effects if calcium channel blockers are taken together with beta blockers. They may enhance one another, so the combination must be carefully watched.

Nifedipine was considered a highly successful drug launch, with sales leveling off at over five million dollars per month. Controversies such as this seem to illustrate the economic pressure on drug manufacturers to promote their products.

SIDE EFFECTS

Adverse reactions to the calcium channel blockers, while frequent, generally are not serious. The most common complaints include dizziness, nausea, headache, flushing, and a drop in blood pressure, all of which occur in about ten percent of patients.

Some specialists predict that the calcium blockers will be useful against other heart diseases and the manufacturers liberally estimate that four million heart patients are potential users of the new calcium blocker family of drugs. Since the beta blockers and calcium channel blockers work in different ways, it might be expected that the two will be used together in some difficult cases. The benefits can be cumulative, but so can the toxic side effects.

As might be expected with any profitable new class of drugs, more are on the way. The calcium block lidoflazine to be sold by

Janssen Pharmaceutica as Angex, and nicardipine, to be sold by Syntex Laboratories as Perdipine are two examples. The former has the potential to become one of the safest calcium blockers. Others in the drug pipeline include nitrendipine, nisoldipine, nimodipine, and flunarizine, which is already available abroad. Research continues on yet another one, perhexiline.

Just how all these calcium blockers might differ from one another is not yet clear so it will be some time before your doctor will know which one is best. There is no doubt, however, that as a group, the calcium blockers are a remarkable new class of drugs for the heart.

Nitroglycerin Rides Again

Nitroglycerin, long the mainstay of angina treatment, has recently taken a back seat to the new calcium blockers and beta blockers. These new drugs are not necessarily all that much better than nitroglycerin, but they are able to *prevent* attacks while nitroglycerin's main use was to *stop* an attack in progress.

When given continuously, however, nitroglycerin will help prevent angina attacks. Until recently this was only feasible in the hospital. The development of several new long-acting, continuous, through-the-skin delivery systems promises to re-establish this explosive drug as a major form of treatment.

Three companies currently sell a small, flexible bandage-like skin patch containing nitroglycerin. Once stuck onto the skin, the patch releases nitroglycerin slowly for a minimum of twenty-four hours. Because the drug is released continuously through the skin into the bloodstream, more of it is able to reach the heart before it is destroyed by the liver. The products currently available are Nitro-Dur, Transderm-Nitro, and Nitrodisc. Although each is somewhat different, all are safe, convenient, and reliable.

They seem to have been well accepted, perhaps because of the added convenience they offer and their ability to guard the patient while he or she sleeps. Once the pad containing the drug is stuck to the skin, it takes from half an hour to an hour for the nitroglycerin to start working, which means this type of nitroglycerin cannot begin to compare with the instant results offered by the under-the-tongue variety.

Just how fast and how much of the drug is absorbed through the skin from one of these patches seems to vary from person to person, and doctors have had problems deciding on the right dosage. Physicians experienced with the use of the pads also suggest varying the place on the skin where they are attached each time. One other drawback is that the pads are rather expensive compared to other forms of the drug.

The Magic of Beta Blockers

It has become clear after fifteen years of use in the United States, that a group of heart drugs called beta blockers are one of those revolutionary advances that come along so rarely. There is general agreement that the introduction of the first such drug, propranolol, has been the single most important therapeutic advance in the treatment of heart disease. The number of available beta blocker drugs is growing and so is the list of their potential uses, including protecting people from second heart attacks.

Six of these drugs are now available by prescription in the United States and the number is likely to increase. In addition to propranolol (Inderal), the others are nadolol (Corgard), timolol (Blocadren), metoprolol (Lopressor), atenolol (Tenormin), and pindolol (Visken). Propranolol is the most widely used, and it has held the lofty position of the number two selling drug in the country.

This group of drugs has achieved popularity because of its safety and effectiveness against a variety of problems not limited to the heart. All beta blockers have been shown useful against high blood pressure and some also work against angina pectoris, abnormal heartbeats, migraine headaches, and chronic glaucoma, which involves increased pressure on the eye. That list may grow to include uses against alcohol withdrawal and even anxiety.

The benefits of beta blockers come from their ability to block the activation of certain nerve sites in the body called beta receptors. Normally, these nerves are switched on by chemicals released from nerve endings. Those chemicals are called norepinephrine and epinephrine, more commonly known as adrenaline.

The result of this blocking effect is a drop in the activity of certain muscles. That in turn counteracts the abnormal activity that goes along with the diseases the drug is being used against.

Scientists have discovered that there are really two kinds of beta receptors called beta-1 and beta-2. Some of the drugs block both, while other beta blocker drugs are more selective and only work against the beta-1 receptors. Which ones should be used depends on the individual and whether or not the person is susceptible to various side effects.

Most of the benefits come from blocking the beta-1 sites. In fact, blocking the beta-2 sites is potentially dangerous since it can worsen lung problems such as asthma. However, in actual practice, doctors still most often prescribe the drugs that block both beta-1 *and* beta-2 sites. Why? Partly because they are the drugs that have been around the longest (and doctors are most familiar with them), and partly because most people are not susceptible to the potential adverse effects. The two available drugs that block only beta-1 sites are metoprolol and atenolol. The others block both types of receptors.

The greater accuracy of metoprolol and atenolol give them some advantages. They can be tried cautiously on asthmatics, while the others should not. Caution is still suggested because they may not leave the beta-2 sites entirely alone and the worsening of respiratory problems has been noted in some patients. All the beta blockers must also be used cautiously in people suffering from congestive heart failure.

Side Effects

In addition to the possible lung problems and worsening of congestive heart failure, there are some other significant side effects that can go along with use of the beta blockers. If these drugs are being used to control high blood pressure, they should never be stopped suddenly. That can lead to sudden, life-threatening increases in blood pressure. If the drug must be discontinued, it should be done gradually.

Other less serious side effects of beta blockers include dizziness, fatigue, nausea, curbed sexual desire, and cold fingers. For the most part, these should be minor and often disappear with time.

Since so many Americans run for sport, there is another warning that should be sounded. Some heart specialists have been saying that beta blocker drugs can be dangerous for runners because of the effect they have in slowing the heart rate. The reduction in output from the heart could inhibit the flow of blood (and oxygen) to the muscles. A suggested alternative for controlling high blood pressure in people who run might be alpha blocker drugs, which work differently by making the blood vessels enlarge rather than slowing the heart, a result that would seem to be more in tune with the rigors of running.

Differences Among Beta Blockers

When new beta blocker drugs hit the market, they are usually touted as having some kind of significant advantage. However, their differences are usually minor and their therapeutic benefits are virtually identical. Still, this is not always the case. Both na-dolol and pindolol lack the ability to treat abnormal heartbeats and thus cannot always be used interchangeably with propranolol. An-other potentially significant difference that sets nadolol and atenolol apart from the others is that these two drugs stay in the body longer and need only be taken once a day. That could be a big plus for people who have trouble remembering when to take their medica-tion. But there may be a trade-off for that benefit—at least with nadolol—since side effects may be more frequent.

So far, timolol is the only beta blocker that is available in a form that can be used to treat the eye, making it the only one used against glaucoma. It may be purchased under the brand name Timoptic. Recently, a major clinical study in Norway turned up another benefit of timolol. The study showed that an oral prepa-ration of the drug could reduce the chances of death by nearly forty percent for up to three years following a heart attack.

Timolol had been available for oral use in Europe for several years before it was recently approved for use by this route in the United States. Since timolol is the only drug that has been proven to prevent some deaths after heart attacks, it is the only one of the beta blockers specifically approved for this purpose. With the possible exception of atenolol, the similarities among the other beta blockers makes it likely that they will also be shown to have this effect.

The usefulness—not to mention the proven profit potential—to the manufacturers of beta blockers means others will undoubtedly be available before long. A few candidates are presented in the accompanying table. Whether these or others like them turn out to be better than what is already available remains to be seen.

Available Beta Blockers

Generic Name	Trade Name
propranolol	Inderal
nadolol	Corgard
timolol	Blocadren
pindolol	Visken
metoprolol	Lopressor
atenolol	Tenormin

Beta Blockers Under Study

Generic Name	Generic Name
sotalol	alprenolol
acebutalol	bufuralol
betaxolol	bunolol
carteolol	inpea
celiprolol	oxprenolol
cetamolol	penbutolol
esmolol	toliprolol

Congestive Heart Failure: New Drugs Keep the Beat

By the time you reach age seventy, your heart will have beat more than 2.5 billion times, without ever having rested for a full second. While we usually take the heart's incredible durability for granted, the need for that continuous beating means that anything less than perfect performance could be serious or even fatal.

The most common of the potential heart diseases is congestive heart failure, and until recently there has been little real improvement in drugs to treat it for nearly two hundred years. Two new drugs, amrinone and sulmazol, are likely to receive government approval.

The leader has been amrinone, which the FDA gave a "fast track" through the giant federal drug approval bureaucracy. This means the FDA was initially impressed with the drug's possibilities and felt it deserved a boost.

Congestive heart failure affects over three million people in the United States. The problem begins with a fluid buildup in the lungs due to the heart's inability to pump enough blood through the lungs to carry the fluid away. The congestion makes breathing difficult. Some of the other major symptoms of congestive heart failure include excessive fluid retention, shortness of breath, fatigue, and extreme weakness. What happens is that the heart muscle has weakened to the point where it is unable to pump blood effectively through the body.

Two kinds of drugs are generally used to treat patients with failing hearts. One group includes digitalis (the dried leaf of the digitalis or foxglove plant) and related products. Digitalis is a powerful substance and works by increasing the force with which the heart contracts.

The second drug group, called vasodilators, relax the blood vessels, making the heart's job easier.

The mainstays of congestive heart drug therapy are the cardiac glycosides, of which digitalis is one. They have been used since the time of the ancient Egyptians, but it was not until a book on foxglove appeared in 1785 that medical people noticed a link between the digitalis plant and a positive response to congestive heart failure. Digitalis, the active ingredient in foxglove, is available today in a purified form, along with other chemically related products.

Digitalis is a very effective drug but it is also quite toxic. A lethal dose could be only two or three times the effective dose. The new drugs are far less toxic and just as effective as digitalis.

The way both amrinone and sulmazol work, and their side effects, are completely different from digitalis. Although this mechanism of action is not entirely clear, amrinone and sulmazol seem to alter calcium transport in the heart, thus improving the efficiency with which the heart contracts.

Amrinone (Inocor) is being developed by Sterling Drug Inc., which claims the drug will be used in both oral form and by injection. The company says the drug acts directly on the failing heart, inducing it to pump more forcefully. It also has some vasodilator properties, Sterling says, that lighten the workload on the heart, and make its pumping job easier.

Taken orally, the drug takes effect from within thirty minutes to two hours (according to initial testing) and lasts from four to seven hours after a single dosage. Some test subjects took the drug for up to three years without developing tolerance to it. Taken intravenously, the drug reaches peak effectiveness from within six minutes to an hour, according to Sterling.

However, some significant side effects have been reported. They include liver damage, a reduced number of platelets (an essential blood element), abnormal heartbeats, and stomach disorders when the drug is taken orally. Those gastrointestinal problems can include nausea, vomiting, stomach cramps, digestive disturbances, hiccups, and diarrhea. In drug trials, between five and ten percent of the patients stopped using the drug because of those reactions.

Still, compared to digitalis, those side effects are not all that alarming. The benefits seem to outweigh the risks of not treating this life-threatening problem.

Sulmazol, while further from approval in the United States, looks to be just as effective in increasing the force of the heartbeat. It, too, can be given orally and thus far has not displayed serious side effects. In Europe it will be marketed under the name Vardax.

Stopping A Heart Attack in its Tracks

Suddenly you feel a crushing weight on your chest. There is pain, you cannot breathe, and you feel nauseated. You may be suffering a heart attack, as more than two people do *every minute* in the United States.

What medical treatment can you expect? Not so many years ago you might have received little more than instructions to take it easy and stay in bed for a month or more.

Today, treatment for heart attacks is one of the most sophisticated aspects of modern medicine and includes more and better types of drugs, a number of which appear to be effective in lessening the risk of the patient having subsequent heart attacks.

But what can be done in the first few hours after a heart attack begins? At many major medical centers around the United States, an aggressive new technique is being tested which actually dissolves the blood clot blocking an artery in the heart. It is this blockage that causes the symptoms of a heart attack.

A cardiologist (heart specialist) threads a tube into the blocked heart artery and then injects an enzyme intended to dissolve the clot. The most widely used enzymes are streptokinase (known by the trade name Streptase) and urokinase (known by the trade names Abbokinase and Breokinase).

Urokinase received a big boost in 1981 when it became the first human enzyme to be cloned by the new gene splicing techniques. The leading genetic engineering company Genentech Inc., produced two forms of urokinase, which may someday help alleviate the prohibitively high cost of producing it naturally, by extraction from human urine and kidneys.

For the first time, these drugs may give doctors the ability to stop a heart attack already in progress. Streptokinase can apparently liquefy an attack-causing clot within an hour. The drug has been around for several years, for use against blood clots elsewhere in the body, but only in mid-1982 was it approved by the FDA for use in heart attack cases. The process using these enzymes goes by several different names; thrombolysis, reperfusion, and recanalization. It seems to work about eighty percent of the time.

In most patients, blood begins flowing again through the artery after the clot is dissolved. The hope is that oxygen will arrive at the heart tissue in time to prevent permanent damage. While this treatment has proved safe and effective in a number of test cases, there is still no solid evidence that patients receiving streptokinase and urokinase by this route live longer than patients given more conventional therapies.

Because the treatment is so new, details of the process are still being worked out. Also, no one yet knows all of the adverse effects that might go along with these enzymes. Patients may face the risk of excessive bleeding that could limit the drug's use in some cases. Since streptokinase is a protein foreign to the body, allergic reactions are a real danger for patients. Urokinase, a human enzyme, does not suffer from this limitation, but it is so expensive that streptokinase is usually used anyway.

Since heart attacks generally last twelve to twenty-four hours, with about half of the heart cells which die succumbing in the first few hours, this treatment must be started as rapidly as possible. Many doctors think it is only beneficial if administered in the first three hours after a heart attack begins.

Streptokinase has been used in Europe to treat heart attacks for several years and both streptokinase and urokinase are available in the United States to dissolve clots in the lung. A recent American study has shown that streptokinase can decrease deaths after heart attacks by about twenty percent. However, these patients received the drug intravenously and there is evidence that this has induced excess bleeding.

The major new advance made in the United States for treating heart attacks with these agents was to infuse the enzyme directly into the blocked artery. This not only put the enzyme where it was needed, but allowed a dramatic reduction in the dose, which should decrease adverse side effects.

Some doctors are quite enthusiastic about this method while others advocate a cautious approach. To complicate matters, physicians should obtain written, informed consent from the patient before using this method. The obvious difficulty in getting written consent from a person suffering a heart attack has slowed development of the therapy.

Even if it proves to be as effective as current studies show, there will be one more problem to overcome: There aren't enough trained cardiologists to administer the procedure to the estimated six hundred thousand people who suffer heart attacks each year. Because of the critical time factor, moving the patient would involve unacceptable delays.

Streptokinase is not the only enzyme that may be helping heart attack victims. Three studies in England have suggested that a purified enzyme called hyaluronidase can reduce the amount of heart damage caused by a heart attack if it is injected early enough. Just why it works is not yet known, but it may be connected to the enzyme's ability to eat the substance blocking the blood vessel. The enzyme has appeared to be quite safe in most patients, although more study will be needed to prove it can really be helpful.

With a bit more time, heart attacks may no longer be the killers they are today.

Preventing Heart Attacks and Keeping the Heart in Rhythm

In addition to stopping attacks in progress, today's treatment has also moved toward preventing the second or third heart attacks that survivors of a first attack often experience. Aspirin is just one of the drugs showing promise (see Chapter 17, *Aspirin: A Tablet a Day May Keep More Than Headaches Away* for more on this), along with several others that like aspirin inhibit the clumping of tiny blood cells called platelets.

One example is a drug called sulfinpyrazone, currently available under the Geigy trade name Anturane, which is used to treat gout. A recent study concluded that sulfinpyrazone can prevent the sudden deaths of some people who have recently suffered a heart attack. However, there's been a lot of controversy surrounding that report, and some people believe the drug cannot really help.

It may be a moot question, since other drugs that can help prevent heart attacks in different ways are also being developed. One promising candidate is ticlopidine, which, while still in the early stages of development, has given encouraging results.

Keeping the heart in good working order once a heart attack has taken place is yet another target of new drugs. The damage done to the heart muscle during an attack usually causes the heart to beat abnormally even after the patient has recovered. The abnormal beats can easily be detected by an electrocardiogram, and this is one of the ways to tell if a person has had a heart attack. Sometimes the heartbeats will return to normal; sometimes they will not, but it will not cause any problems; in other cases the abnormalities grow severe enough to result in death. Several drugs are already available to help control this, but none of them work all the time. New drugs to help fill this gap currently under development include ecainide, flecainide, aprindine, mexiletine, tocainide, and cibenzoline.

Encainide seems to be the standout among this group, and the FDA is also considering approving flecainide, which carries the brand name Tambocar.

Amiodarone, another one of these drugs, is very effective and has been available in Europe since 1961. But it probably will never be approved for use in the United States because it has been linked to a serious lung disorder called pulmonary fibrosis.

Hypertension: New Drugs to Control High Blood Pressure

There may seem to be a constant influx of new high blood pressure medications known as antihypertensives, but true advances against this insidious disease are rare. In the past, development of the thiazide diuretics, and introduction of the beta blockers were big steps against hypertension (high blood pressure). Now there are a few new products that approach blood pressure control in a unique way. Someday they may also prove to be major advances.

Individuals with problem high blood pressure that has not responded well to drug treatment or who have developed unacceptable side effects with other drugs now have an alternative. A new drug, captopril (also known by the trade name Capoten) is now being marketed and works inside the body in a totally different way than the other drugs used to treat hypertension.

For many years, drugs used to treat hypertension fell into three groups: water pills (diuretics); blood vessel relaxers (vasodilators); and drugs that alter the nervous system. Medications from these three groups are often used in combinations to best achieve a normal blood pressure. Although they are usually quite effective, many of them cause unpleasant side effects and some patients have not responded well to the treatment.

This new drug, however, works in a different way—by preventing the body from producing a chemical (angiotensin) which acts to elevate the blood pressure. The result in most people is a modest but sustained decrease in blood pressure. Since it attacks the problem from a different angle, however, captopril can be used with other drugs to get a better overall result.

By using this new drug, the required doses of the others can be reduced and therefore, the unpleasant side effects can also be proportionately lessened.

Hypertension is a common disorder affecting 10 to 15 percent of white adults and 20 to 30 percent of black adults in the United States. Doctors are able to pinpoint a cause in only about one out of every ten cases. The remainder are called essential hypertension which, while not curable, can be controlled with drugs.

High blood pressure is a disease in which there are usually no obvious symptoms. Except for an acute hypertensive crisis, which is immediately life-threatening, high blood pressure is dangerous because it slowly damages the heart over a period of time. This has helped make heart disease the leading cause of death in the United States today.

People with high blood pressure can usually bring it down to acceptable levels with the drugs available, thus greatly diminishing the high risk of heart disease. But the lack of outward symptoms is the big problem. People are too often reluctant to take medicine which, because of its side effects, makes them feel worse than they felt before. By the time the symptoms do begin to show themselves, the heart damage is far advanced and irreversible.

While most of the drug side effects will diminish or disappear with time, many people are not willing to wait, so they stop taking the medication prematurely. As with many other afflictions, the drugs can only treat the symptoms of high blood pressure and not the disease itself. But unlike many other diseases, treating the symptoms of high blood pressure is enough to prevent further heart damage and the only requirement is to stay on the medication.

According to the drug firm Squibb, Capoten is a drug that can help control blood pressure without many of the usual side effects of blood pressure drugs. The drug company says there is no blood potassium deficiency (hypokalemia), and no slowdown in the heartbeat. And, says Squibb, Capoten can be used when other high blood pressure-related diseases are also present, such as congestive heart failure, diabetes mellitus, liver disease, and bronchospastic disease.

The FDA has actually approved Capoten as an adjunct treatment for patients with congestive heart failure. In people who are not helped with digitalis and diuretics, the addition of Capoten can often be of great benefit.

Beware, however, since some severe side effects can go along with the use of Capoten. The most frequent are skin rashes and the impairment of the sense of taste. Although reversible, this loss of taste takes place in about seven percent of patients taking the drug. Rashes occur even more frequently—about ten percent of the time—usually during the first four weeks of taking the drug.

Potential effects on the kidney and bone marrow have also been reported with this drug, but overall, if it is used properly under a doctor's direction, it is a good addition to the list of other hypertension drugs.

As might be expected with a successful new drug, similar products are waiting in the wings. Merck, Sharp & Dohme is working on enalapril, another chemical which works much the same as captopril. If this new product turns out to have fewer side effects than captopril, it could do even better.

OTHER NEW CHOICES

The most potent oral blood pressure drug available is minoxidil (Loniten). But the price for that potency is some potent side effects, which together have made this a fall-back drug if nothing else seems to be working. Minoxidil works by directly relaxing the blood vessels. One of the drug's unusual side effects, disconcerting to many patients, is that it stimulates hair growth. Unfortunately, when taken orally, minoxidil is not particular about *where* it stimulates the growth of hair, or in which sex.

Other drugs which relax blood vessels are currently being worked on. Nisoldipine and nitrendipine are only two examples of this group. Although no more effective than minoxidil, they work by a different mechanism and the hope is to eliminate some of the side effects.

The effectiveness of yet another antihypertensive drug, prazosin is just now being appreciated. Prazosin, sold under the trade name Minipress by the drug company Pfizer Inc., is currently the only drug of its kind on the market. It is considered an alpha blocker and it prevents blood vessels from constricting. When blood vessels constrict, blood pressure is raised, like squeezing a garden hose.

Minipress, the manufacturer claims, goes after the main problem—the constriction of the blood vessels. Drugs that affect the heart, the company says, do not do anything about the source of the problem. As Pfizer trumpets in its advertising to doctors, "Hypertension is *not* a heart disease." Minipress can cause fainting and other side effects including dizziness (10.3 percent of the time), headache (7.8 percent of the time), and drowsiness (7.6 percent of the time). Abbott Laboratories is working on an improved relative of this drug, called terazosin, which should be available by the mid-1980s. Pfizer is studying others, such as doxazosin and timazosin (Cardouar).

As these alpha blocker drugs become more widely used, it is becoming clear that they can also be highly useful second line drugs for blood pressure cases that do not respond to the thiazide diuretics (water pills) that are most often tried first because they are safe, effective for most people, and inexpensive. People who cannot take beta blockers because of asthma, congestive heart failure, or diabetes, might be able to take an alpha blocker.

The greatest concern with alpha blockers is the possibility of a sudden drop in blood pressure, as sometimes happens when prazosin therapy is first started. The problem is usually overcome with repeated doses, but individuals must be closely watched, and should be forewarned of possible dizziness, fainting, and heart palpitations.

Some of the problems with alpha and beta blocking drugs may be overcome with a unique new product called labetalol which blocks *both* alpha and beta receptors. This drug, which will be sold by Schering as Normodyne and by Glaxo as Trandate, is the only one which can be used in both a hypertensive emergency and for followup to maintain a stable blood pressure. Labetalol also has little effect on heart rate in contrast to most beta blockers and seems to eliminate at least some of the need for the use of diuretics along with alpha or beta blockers to adequately lower blood pressure.

Another antihypertensive drug recently approved is guanabenz acetate, marketed by Wyeth Labs as Wytensin. Guanabenz combines the chemistry of two older antihypertensive drugs: guanethidine (Ismelin) and clonidine (Catapres). Although how it works is not completely clear, it seems to act by stimulating sites in the brain called alpha receptors which then lower the blood pressure. Guanabenz becomes the third product available that works this way, joining clonidine and alpha methyldopa (Aldomet).

The most agreeable aspect of guanabenz is its mild side effects —especially when compared to Aldomet. Sodium (salt) retention, seen with related drugs, is not a problem with guanabenz. There is also no clinical evidence of liver damage. The adverse reactions that are seen include dry mouth, drowsiness, dizziness, weakness, and headache. While not severe, they occur in up to fifty-three percent of the patients taking Wytensin, and are troublesome enough that fifteen percent switch to other drugs.

Since it is so new, Wytensin's exact role in the treatment of high blood pressure is not yet clear. It may be used alone or combined with other drugs, and may help control mild to severe hypertension. While not a major new drug, it does appear to improve on existing antihypertensive drugs.

Lofexidine is another blood pressure drug that works on the brain. It is not available yet in the United States but has been on the market in Europe under the brand name Lofetensin, and will be sold in the United States by Merrell-Dow Pharmaceuticals as Loxacor. It seems to work much like clonidine. Importantly, however, it has far less of a sedative effect than does clonidine. The tired feeling that many people get from using clonidine has been a major problem with that drug. Other newcomers include guanadrel sulfate (Hylorel) from Pennwalt Corporation, and urapidil from Marion Laboratories. Urapidil is a fascinating compound, and the first to combine two methods of lowering blood pressure. It should be available in the late 1980s.

RISK REDUCTION QUESTIONED

A ten-year study, the largest ever done on risks associated with heart disease, has raised new questions about standard medical thinking on heart disease and high blood pressure. Results of the massive study, financed by the National Heart, Lung and Blood Institute, were first announced in September 1982. They immediately caused a stir.

In particular, the finding which raised eyebrows questioned the safety of using thiazide diuretics, the most popular blood pressure drugs, on specific groups of people. Researchers were surprised to find that men with abnormal heart rhythms (abnormal electrocardiogram readings) who also were being treated with thiazide diuretics for high blood pressure, actually had a higher death rate than other men considered at risk of heart disease.

That finding led to speculation that these diuretics cause different bodily responses in people with abnormal heartbeats. Since over five million Americans are estimated to suffer from abnormal heart rhythms, this question is of more than passing interest. But the results of this study, sometimes called the "Mr. Fit Study," were not conclusive about the actual cause of this higher rate, and another study has been planned.

One reason such conclusions could not be drawn was that during the ten years of this study, the entire United States population had a decreased risk of heart attacks, presumably due to changing lifestyles and new drugs. The investigators had to look for larger decreases on top of an overall decrease in order to find benefits with the drugs they were testing.

The original $115 million study, involving 12,866 men considered to be high risk because of high blood pressure, smoking habits, or high cholesterol, was carried out at twenty-two medical centers throughout the United States and Canada. The study did seem to confirm the dramatic lessening of coronary risk that can be achieved by changes in lifestyle among high-risk individuals. Stopping smoking, eating less fat, and lowering cholesterol intake can cut the risk of coronary deaths in half, according to the results of the massive study. It also appeared that except for people with abnormal heartbeats, lowering the blood pressure with diuretics was beneficial.

DISPUTE OVER POTASSIUM SUPPLEMENT

It has been known for years that taking thiazide diuretic drugs can lower the level of potassium in a person's body, which in turn could aggravate abnormal heartbeats. Doctors, worried about the depletion of potassium, have long prescribed potassium supplements at the same time. The supplements were mostly foul-tasting liquids—a problem that has changed with the introduction of controlled-release potassium tablets such as Slow-K, K-Tab, Micro-K, and Kaon-Cl that have made it much safer and more pleasant to take potassium. An alternative has been the use of diuretics that do not cause this loss of blood potassium. Called potassium-sparing diuretics, the newest one is amiloride, sold as Midamor. Eating bananas is another alternative, but you would have to consume a half-dozen of them every day to get the amount of potassium that is lost.

But now, researchers are saying that taking the potassium supplements may be unnecessary, and perhaps even worse than living with the deficiency. Doctors have been writing about 7.5 million prescriptions for potassium supplements each year to go along with the ten million prescriptions for potassium-sparing diuretic drugs. The money spent on these drugs exceeds two hundred fifty million dollars.

The dispute over potassium supplements grows in part out of the lack of any studies showing that small decreases in potassium levels in the body are dangerous (except for people taking digitalis). On the other hand, too much potassium has been linked to cardiac arrest. The lack of scientific justification for taking potassium supplements calls for more studies and in the meantime caution in using them.

TREATMENT HAS COME A LONG WAY

Since the 1950s, when many medical people actually thought hypertension was beneficial (so much the better to pump blood to the extremities), drugs available to treat it have made massive strides. Back then, when doctors knew little or nothing about high blood pressure, one of the major alternatives to treating it was putting the patient on a rice diet.

That has all changed, of course, and the trend today is toward treating even mild cases of high blood pressure, since, left untreated, hypertension can dramatically increase your chances of later developing other heart problems. With an estimated sixty million Americans affected by hypertension, that will be a mighty challenge to antihypertensive drugs, but one it appears they can handle.

29

HEPATITIS B VACCINE BEGINS ITS WORK

It has its work cut out for it, but at least a new vaccine designed to fight the most serious type of hepatitis can finally begin its task. The vaccine against hepatitis B, which became commercially available in the United States in mid-1982, took a long time to get onto the market, even after its approval by the government back in late 1981.

Why the delay? Because the hepatitis B vaccine, called Heptavax-B, takes an incredibly long time to make and test—sixty-five weeks in all, according to manufacturer Merck, Sharp & Dohme. No doubt that is also a factor in making the stuff so expensive. A three-dose series, which is necessary for it to work, runs about $100, or $30 to $35 per dosage.

But unlike polio or measles vaccines, Heptavax-B is not recommended for everyone. This is because exposure to the hepatitis virus is only significant to certain groups of people, and it is these at-risk individuals who should be vaccinated. Some of those at-risk groups include: health care personnel (the risk for doctors is about one in five), dentists and dental hygienists, patients and staff who receive or work with blood and blood components, active homosexuals, family and friends of hepatitis B victims, drug addicts, staff and residents of mental institutions and prisons, and some ethnic groups such as Alaskan Eskimos and Indochinese.

An estimated two hundred thousand people in the United States get hepatitis B each year. More than four thousand will die and thousands more may be bedridden for weeks or months and suffer permanent liver damage from the disease. People in Third World nations suffer far more from this disease, and it is there that a vaccine can be of even greater importance, although the cost looks like a problem.

In the United States there is another group estimated at up to eight hundred thousand people who, although they do not have an active form of the disease, are carriers nonetheless and may be unwittingly spreading it. These modern-day Typhoid Marys are actually essential for the production of the new vaccine.

As with most viral infections, there are no drugs that can cure hepatitis. The challenge has been to come up with a vaccine to immunize people against the disease, much as medical science has done with smallpox, polio, measles, and mumps. But the hepatitis B virus is a bit quirky in that it will not grow in an egg or a cell culture like most other viruses. And growing it that way in a laboratory was considered essential to manufacturing a vaccine.

Ironically, carriers of the disease finally provided the solution. Their bodies release large amounts of viral surface antigens—substances which lead the body to produce antibodies—into their bloodstreams. Once researchers discovered that those antigens could stimulate an immune response in other people, the route to the vaccine was clear, if not easy. But the manufacturer had better be extremely careful in purifying these antibody producers to make sure the virus is totally inactivated. If not, a vaccinated individual could be accidentally infected with hepatitis.

Merck, Sharp & Dohme is now producing the vaccine in large quantity, using blood from hepatitis carriers. Testing has shown it to be nearly ninety-six percent effective in persons receiving the recommended three shots; the second dose coming a month after the first, and the third dose six months after the first.

A possible but as yet unproven benefit of the vaccine could be to diminish the number of people contracting liver cancer, since the hepatitis virus and development of liver cancer have been closely linked in recent medical literature. It could make Heptavax-B the first vaccine against cancer. If this particular type of liver cancer is indeed caused by or associated with the hepatitis B virus, immunized people could be resistant to this cancer.

The testing of Heptavax-B turned up very little in the way of adverse reactions or side-effects. Some soreness where the injection was made is common, and there have been some cases of fever reported. But so far in the early stages, no serious or long-term side-effects have cropped up.

The hepatitis B vaccine is surely good news, but it is not a cure or treatment for the disease itself. Heptavax-B is of no use if given after hepatitis develops. It is also of no use if the patient is infected with hepatitis A, or other agents that can produce the disease.

Depending on how popular the vaccine is, there could be shortages of it because of the lengthy manufacturing and testing process. But now that it is finally here, it promises to be a lifesaver.

30

HERPES:
THE DEFIANT EPIDEMIC

Herpes has become one of the toughest and most widespread medical problems the United States has yet faced. Its rise to domination is now well known, even though doctors all over the country were failing to recognize it up until the late 1970s.

Precise figures are hard to come by since doctors are not required to report herpes cases as they are for the more serious venereal diseases. But estimates by the Center for Disease Control in Atlanta put the number of genital herpes cases in America at nearly twenty million. Well over one thousand people are believed to contract a new case of the disease *every day.*

Many people continue to believe that curing a venereal disease (VD) is a simple matter because of the tremendous success of penicillin and other antibiotics. Those people would be right if the VD field were limited to bacterial infections such as gonorrhea and syphillis. But it is not.

The world's most widespread and one of the oldest venereal diseases is herpes, and it is caused by a virus, not a bacterium. Fighting viruses has been a persistent leak in the medical dike of drugs. (Also see Chapter 43, *Viral Infections*).

For herpes, there is no cure yet, nor does it look like one is immediately forthcoming. A drug that can kill this wily virus and rid the human body of the disease entirely may be too much to hope for at this time. Medical science has a long way to go.

There are other steps that will help, however. The mobilization of research against herpes is helping to bring about a medical revolution in the battle against viruses.

Public awareness of herpes came with a crushing swiftness. We are still finding out more about it all the time. It came as a shock, for instance, when it was recently noted that herpes simplex 1— oral herpes which is responsible for cold sores—can be transferred to the genital areas by physical contact. The herpes virus makes itself known in several forms, and is responsible for such human ailments as chickenpox, shingles, and cold sores, in addition to the genital variety caused by herpes simplex 2.

The symptoms of genital herpes begin mildly as a tingling or burning sensation of the skin which rapidly becomes a rash. This is followed by lesions which are highly infectious. These painful sores can last up to three weeks (although later outbreaks usually stay around only a few days), accompanied by fever, aches, and discomfort.

The virus itself never goes away. Since medicine does not yet know how to kill it, once contracted, you have it for life, or until a cure is found. After an acute attack of herpes the virus goes into hiding somewhere in the body, entering a dormant state from which it can reawaken at just about any time for unknown reasons. It almost seems like something from a science fiction horror show.

From a medical standpoint, herpes is not as serious as other venereal diseases which can cause blindness, sterility, and death. However, there can be serious consequences in pregnancies. Babies born to mothers with active herpes outbreaks run a high risk of contracting the disease, and many babies will either die or suffer serious brain damage.

As for adults, it is not going to kill them. But then again, they are not going to kill it either—at least not yet.

Although herpes is a virus, it is not like many other viruses (such as the ones that cause the flu or colds). This one continues to live on in the human body after the initial attack subsides. Scientists do not know how or why the herpes virus reawakens from its inactive state. Once they figure that out, perhaps they will be able to come up with a drug to stop it.

In the meantime, a product to help relieve initial outbreaks sooner and perhaps cut down on their frequency is already available.

ONE OF THE FASTEST DRUG APPROVALS EVER

It became one of the quickest drug approvals on record when the FDA announced late in March 1982 that it was giving the green light to acyclovir—the first drug to effectively treat *initial* outbreaks of genital herpes. That alone signified recognition by the FDA of the growing herpes epidemic.

The drug is available by prescription under the trade name Zovirax. It is a creamy ointment and remains the only FDA-approved anti-herpes drug in the United States. Acyclovir was developed and is marketed by the Burroughs Wellcome Co.

Keep in mind, however, that Zovirax is *not* a cure by any stretch of the imagination. It is a treatment, and although expectations were high when it was first introduced, it has turned out to have limited use.

Applied topically, acyclovir speeds the rate of healing of the herpes lesions. That healing effect is useful since it lessens the time the virus can be transmitted to others, as well as comforts the patient. Shortly after the drug went on the market, however, a report appeared in the *New England Journal of Medicine* indicating that topical acyclovir is not effective in treating outbreaks of herpes beyond the first one. That was a severe blow to millions who had hoped for a product to offer, at last, some continued relief. Fortunately, the report did verify the effectiveness of the drug used topically on people suffering their first, and usually most severe, herpes episode.

The FDA has recommended that doctors not prescribe acyclovir for anything other than first-time outbreaks of herpes.

The *New England Journal of Medicine* study also showed that acyclovir cannot help reduce the number of times the herpes outbreaks will recur.

Nevertheless, there is still much hope for acyclovir. It appears that if the drug is given orally, or intravenously, it is much more effective. The intravenous form is now available and the oral form should follow soon. Although it is still only indicated for initial outbreaks of genital herpes, it can be used against other forms of herpes that attack other sites in the body.

A HERPES VACCINE AND OTHER DRUG TREATMENTS

Going hand in hand with the search for drugs to cure herpes is a big effort to develop a vaccine that can prevent people from getting it in the first place. The Lederle Laboratories division of American Cyanamid Company has joined up with Molecular Genetics Inc. in one such effort to develop a commercial vaccine against herpes simplex 1 and 2. These firms are using genetic engineering technology to develop the vaccine. Even if they are successful, it will be years before something would be available to the public. Human tests of two other herpes vaccines have begun in the United States, although the results of these, and others sure to follow, are not yet in. Interferon, one of the potential drugs to be used against herpes, is also years away from becoming commercially available.

Another drug, isoprinosine, may also be effective against herpes. This drug, produced by Newport Pharmaceuticals, is already available in nearly sixty countries, but not in the United States. It seems to work by stimulating the body's own defenses against the virus, thus enabling you to fight it off. Attempts are being made to test and approve this drug for use against herpes in the United States. Based on experience with isoprinosine in other countries, there are claims that it can cut down on the number of times the herpes lesions will reappear. This is no cure either, but if this approach (building up the body's immune system) works, it could give herpes sufferers some chance to limit flare-ups. (See Chapter 43, *Viral Infections: Struggling Against the Beguiling Virus* for more details on isoprinosine.)

As with other viruses, many people think the first effective drug against herpes will be one of the immunostimulants like isoprinosine that boost your body's own natural defenses against the virus.

Other more powerful drugs to stop the lesions once they appear are in the development stages and may be on the market by the late 1980s. Enzo Biochem Inc., for example, is testing an interferon preparation that seems to work against herpes. And recently a Swedish research team reported on a drug called foscavir, which they claim can reduce herpes symptoms in as little as one day. Vidarabine, a drug already available to treat other forms of herpes, is also being tested for the venereal disease, while Searle is testing a product known as BVDU and Upjohn is testing one called ABPP (2-amino-5-bromo-6-phenyl-4-pyrimidinol), which increases interferon production.

One additional product waiting in the wings carries the name BIOLF-62. When aimed at genital herpes it seems to be more effective than acyclovir, even though it is chemically similar. When applied topically, BIOLF-62 has been shown to eliminate one thousand times more herpes virus than acyclovir. Once again, however, it is not a cure. It is simply another improvement toward a product that can provide rapid relief from the symptoms of the disease. The drug is still in the experimental stages and will have to undergo more testing before it can reach the market.

Since many herpes sufferers report that nerves often play a role in bringing on attacks, it may be that chemical changes brought on by nerve impulses (the herpes virus resides with the nerves) can cause the virus to activate itself. Other contributors in bringing about outbreaks can be menstruation, sexual activity, and even sunlight. This, in turn, leads many people to believe that herpes outbreaks can be suppressed without drugs, literally by the power of positive thinking. By eliminating the stress that contributes to recurrences, herpes sufferers may have a weapon they can use themselves.

31

INTERFERON: FLASH GORDON'S MIRACLE CURE COMES DOWN TO EARTH

Not many people paid attention at the time, but the excitement over interferon began aboard Flash Gordon's comic-strip spaceship somewhere in the galaxy in 1960. Amidst much worry and wringing of hands a great cry goes out from the rocket ship's laboratory: "This could be it," cries the doctor. "Interferon! Hurry!" In the next episode, the patient's fever comes down and the "miracle drug" is declared a success.

All the pieces seemed to fit. Even the sound of the word interferon has a futuristic ring to it, like some exotic new space age substance ready to step in and cure many of man's illnesses.

As we entered the decade of the 1980s, genetic engineering brought interferon back into the headlines, this time for real. The American public was told interferon could do just about anything. We were promised the moon, but we have not yet taken delivery.

Interferon is probably not all that it was cracked up to be a few years ago. But tests of interferon in humans are turning up positive results, and there is still a lot of excitement over interferon's potential uses. Interferons (there are several types) are proteins that appear naturally in the human body in tiny amounts. The substance is thought to be one of the body's first lines of defense against an attacking virus.

When a virus invades one of your cells, the production of interferon is triggered. This interferon spreads to other cells, switching on further production of these antiviral proteins to ward off the virus. It seems to do so by inhibiting the reproduction of viral particles.

Perhaps best of all, however, is that interferon seems to work against all viruses, while antibodies (another of your body's natural defenses) are selective in what they fight.

What this suggested, as far back as 1957 when two British scientists first identified interferon, is that viral infections could be cured simply by giving the patient interferon.

The stumbling block in this scenario has been making the interferon. The problem is this: Interferon is species specific, which is to say that only human interferon will work in humans. This differs from other proteins, such as insulin, that can be transferred from one species to another.

Huge amounts of human blood were required to extract only a tiny amount of rather impure interferon and there was not even enough for researchers to run clinical tests on the drug. That is, until now.

The solution to the availability problem has come from genetic engineering, also known as recombinant DNA technology or, simply, gene splicing. Scientists now transfer the human genetic information responsible for making interferon to other cells that then act as microscopic factories, producing highly pure interferon in large vats. Several pharmaceutical and genetic engineering companies are already doing so, and it appears interferon can be produced in large quantities at a reasonable cost. Prices for the interferon used in clinical tests have already come down tremendously from what they were a short time ago.

Medical centers in the United States, Britain, and other countries are conducting trials of the genetically engineered interferon, as well as interferon that is taken from natural sources. One of the main targets is fighting cancer, although interferon's great potential for use against viral disease is being pursued in tests involving hepatitis, influenza, herpes, and the common cold as well.

Hundreds of experiments in England, using a simple interferon nasal spray or nose drops, have left little doubt that it can stop a cold virus dead in its tracks. Of course this does not mean it will cure a cold *after* it develops, so practical difficulties abound and it is doubtful that interferon could ever be widely used against the common cold. But the fact that it works so well in this case makes turning it against other viral infections look exciting.

One of the biggest hopes for interferon was against cancer, but those results have been discouraging in many cases. It is not turning out to be the big breakthrough in the cancer battle that was anticipated in the early going. It may well join a list of other drugs useful against cancer in a multiple drug attack, but does not seem able to go it alone.

Even though scientists have known about interferon since 1957, they still have much to learn about it, and how it works in the body, including how many kinds of interferon there really are, and which ones will be the most effective against certain diseases. The fact that there are so many varieties is itself a positive discovery, as scientists may find interferons specially tailored to fight specific diseases.

One positive report on interferon says it decreases the severity of chickenpox (a viral disease) in children with cancer. That's important because chickenpox can be life-threatening to kids undergoing chemotherapy. This also serves as further evidence that interferon can be effective against other viral infections.

With so few antiviral drugs available, that would be a major medical advancement. But although interferon has received a big publicity buildup, it still has a distance to go in the long government approval process.

Yet the potential uses for interferon continue to grow. One recent study at the Baylor College of Medicine in Houston suggests that interferon may help halt the recurrence of wart-like growths in the throat that can make talking and breathing difficult. While these growths are rarely cancerous, some patients had to have them surgically removed every two weeks. Interferon offers the first hopeful alternative to this previously grim prognosis.

Side Effects Could Cause Trouble

There has been trouble brewing for interferon. Until recently, these amazing proteins had not come under extensive scrutiny for possible side effects. Most of the attention was on producing more interferon by genetic engineering, and on testing it against viral diseases.

The list of side effects that have now been linked directly to interferon has lengthened considerably. One French study turned up potentially severe effects on the heart—disturbances of heart rhythm, particularly dangerous in people who already have heart problems. Vomiting, diarrhea, inhibition of blood cell formation in the bone marrow, and liver damage are other serious side effects now linked to interferon. The possibility of liver damage is particularly alarming for infants. Studies in newborn rats and mice showed that interferon could cause massive liver damage and even death. This could also be a problem in adults, with long-term use.

Harmful side effects from interferon come somewhat unexpectedly. Since interferon is a natural substance found in the human body, most scientists thought it would turn out to be quite safe. That belief, however, is not correct. It only persisted as long as it did because early interferon samples (before introduction of highly pure genetically engineered interferons) were very impure—up to ninety-nine percent impure—and researchers blamed side effects on the impurities.

So far, although the side effects are causing concern, it is unlikely they are enough to prevent interferon from being used successfully in clinical tests. The side effects are reversible when treatment with interferon is stopped, and the most severe effects seem limited to long-term use. With short-term treatments, the most common side effects include fever and chills, which are not considered serious.

Ralph Nader's Health Research Group has stirred the pot with charges that Hoffmann-LaRoche, a giant drug firm and leading maker of interferon, did not inform investigators using their interferon of possible central nervous system damage. Roche refuted the charge, and an author of the study citing the side effects said the dangers were being overblown.

In addition to Roche's project, another major interferon production and testing venture involves the drug firm Schering-Plough. Schering is working with the biotechnology firm Biogen, and hopes to market an interferon product by 1985. Hoffmann-LaRoche is working with the leading biotech outfit Genentech. They are testing interferon against several viruses and cancers.

But despite the multimillion dollar efforts, no genetically produced interferon preparation has yet been shown to be safe and effective against any disease. Still, Schering must be confident since the firm has decided to commit over one hundred million dollars to interferon production facilities.

At the same time, all the hoopla over genetically engineered interferon has overshadowed another approach to using interferon against disease. That alternative is an interferon "inducer"—a chemical that stimulates the body to produce interferon on its own more rapidly. An advantage this approach may have is an ability to stimulate interferon production at the site of the problem.

Different chemicals can be used as interferon inducers. One, called poly(I) poly(C), has received the most attention, although other research is focusing on drugs such as acridanone, tilorone, and anthraquinone.

If the obstacles can be overcome, interferon might finally make a positive change in man's ability to fight viruses.

32

MEMORY LOSS: CAN DRUGS STOP IT?

It is not yet possible to buy a drug that will stop an aging person from experiencing memory loss, but it may not be long before that changes.

Excellent results are already being achieved in tests of memory drugs where young and old subjects alike have shown marked improvements in memory. Work remains experimental, but the positive results have shown that at least some memory loss associated with aging can be stopped.

A fading of mental capacity, particularly of memory, is one of the most feared consequences of growing old. For most people, aging seems not to affect their mental abilities, while others develop mild forgetfulness and some people progress to severe and irreversible forms commonly known as senility. Years of research are finally starting to pay off as scientists now better understand what types of drugs will be able to reverse or prevent memory loss.

A widely held view about what causes memory loss involves the chemical acetylcholine which helps transmit nerve impulses in the brain. After many years, this chemical can begin to fail and will not perform up to normal capacity. This failure can result from decreased production of the chemical, from a more rapid rate of destruction, or from a drop in the responsiveness of the nerve to the action of the chemical.

It has been proven, for example, that the brain produces less acetylcholine in people suffering from a severe form of senility called Alzheimer's disease even though there is little wrong with the nerves themselves. Logically you would think all that was necessary would be an increase in the acetylcholine level in the brain of such patients. But there have been few reports of success by doing so.

With other kinds of memory loss, however, the results have been much better. Two basic ways of improving the biochemical workings of memory in the brain are being developed. The simplest and safest method is a special diet containing abundant amounts of a common natural substance called choline. Your body already can make this substance, but foods such as eggs or lecithin can add to it.

The idea is that this choline will be converted to acetylcholine (the memory chemical) in the brain. Some evidence actually shows it works to increase acetylcholine levels, but only one out of seventeen studies conducted on the matter showed a resulting improvement in memory.

A More Promising Method

The outlook may be brighter for increasing acetylcholine levels by the use of drugs or by using a drug that mimics acetylcholine and could stimulate the memory centers. Excellent results have already been achieved with an existing drug called physostigmine. This drug is used to treat glaucoma as well as myasthenia gravis, a disease which causes progressive muscle weakness.

Physostigmine can increase and prolong the action of acetylcholine by preventing its destruction, and subjects who have taken it show marked improvements in memory.

Another substance, arecoline, can mimic the action of acetylcholine and dramatic improvements in memory have been measured with its use. Research on this drug and others related to it remains in the early stages. However, the fact that a drug that mimics acetylcholine works better than those that simply stimulate greater acetylcholine production in the brain could mean that there are other factors involved. That, in turn, could open the door to still other new drugs such as piracetam, pramiracetam, and aniracetam, all of which seem to help the brain work better overall, and may therefore benefit victims of age-related memory loss.

In laboratory animals, combining piracetam with foods containing choline had a dramatic effect on the animals' memories. Even more encouraging, preliminary tests of human patients with Alzheimer's disease produced some improvements.

Other drugs being tested by Lederle Laboratories for the treatment of memory loss include centropheoxine and zasopressin.

The entire area of memory control remains largely a mystery to scientists. Much more research will have to be completed before any product will become available to the public, even for elderly victims of senility. Special care must be taken when dealing with drugs that affect the brain to avoid unwanted side effects. Thus, it will even be longer before memory drugs are available to everyone.

33

MENTAL ILLNESS: DRUG THERAPY AS A DEFENSE AGAINST INSANITY

In this often violent age, the term insanity tends to conjure up visions of people who commit hideous crimes: mass murderers, assassins, and the like. Society loses sight of the more accurate portrait of most of the unfortunate individuals who suffer forms of mental illness, a disease that can disrupt the chemical balance in the brain.

It makes more sense when you realize that the transmission of impulses from one nerve cell to another in the brain is in large part a chemical process, not an electrical one as many people still believe. Scientists are now saying that tiny alterations in those chemicals, called neurotransmitters, can drastically change the way a person behaves and how he or she views the everyday world. Even more important, it may be these tiny chemical changes that actually are behind much of what is known as mental illness, or what a court of law refers to as insanity.

One of today's most widespread psychiatric disorders is severe depression, what the doctor will call endogenous depression. It is different from the "transient" depression caused by life's common events: a death in the family, a marital breakup, problems on the job. People usually get over transient depression with a little time.

But severe or endogenous depression can last months or even years. Often there is no apparent cause either. Sometimes it comes on slowly, other times it hits a person quickly. Suddenly they are unable to function, and they lose themselves in a futureless world of their own. The result is often suicide, a course chosen by up to seventy-five thousand people each year in the United States.

Evidence to back up the idea that chemical changes in the brain are responsible for depression has come from the suicide victims themselves. One recent study discovered that there were actually chemical abnormalities in their brains.

Several kinds of antidepressant drugs have offered one form of help to sufferers of severe depression. Drug therapy has allowed many depressed patients to resume normal or near-normal lives. These drugs, called tricylic antidepressants, seem to work by affecting the metabolism and release of neurotransmitter chemicals in the brain, leading to more normal concentrations of the chemicals.

But the drugs have many limitations. For example, a depressed individual may at the same time also suffer from extreme, irrational anxiety. Doctors have been stymied trying to treat both the depression *and* the anxiety. Older drugs, such as amitriptyline, could only help the depression. Combination products, such as Triavil (perphenazine plus amitriptyline) and Limbitrol (a Valium-related drug plus amitriptyline), tried to go one better by adding tranquilizers. The drug doxepin (Sinequan, Adapin) seemed to be an even better answer by having both effects in a single drug.

But all of these still fell short of the mark. They failed to help about thirty percent of all patients; they were slow, taking up to two weeks to show improvement; they made people drowsy and gave them a dry mouth; and they carried the potential of causing heart damage, even in normal doses.

A Second Generation of Drugs

A second generation of antidepressants with a unique chemical structure and different way of working offer hope for some improvement in fighting these problems. Four of the new drugs are, or soon will be, available in the United States: trazodone, marketed as Desyrel by Mead Johnson and Co.; maprotiline, marketed as Ludiomil by Ciba-Geigy; amoxapine, called Asendin by its manufacturer Lederle Laboratories; and buproprion, sold as Wellbutrin by Burroughs Wellcome.

They do not seem to be any more effective than the older drugs, but at least they have fewer side effects and can work against anxiety associated with depression as well as the depression itself. The lessening of side effects is an important step. Toxicity of the older drugs was such that overdoses could be fatal—an obvious drawback in dealing with depressed, potentially suicidal patients. Trazodone and buproprion in particular seem to have much less effect on the heart, the most dangerous site of side effects. The others seem to offer fewer improvements, although they work a little faster.

Although the general public is mostly unaware of it, these drugs are heavily promoted to the medical community. Slick advertising for the antidepressant/antianxiety drugs, targeted at doctors through medical magazines, often feature pretty pictures of flowers and butterflies. An advertisement for Ludiomil, appearing in numerous medical journals, says that the drug "effectively relieves anxiety associated with depression and may preclude the need for additional tranquilizers . . . it exerts first and foremost an effect on sadness of mood, anxiety, and agitation, without producing undue sedation . . . relief of depression and associated anxiety begins within the first week in some patients." It's all made to sound very nice.

Further information on the drug, provided by the manufacturer, points out that the way Ludiomil works is not precisely known. Extreme caution is advised when the drug is given to someone with heart disease.

Newer drugs in this class, with fewer side effects, are more effective, and better able to control the chemical imbalances causing mental illness. They are likely to be reaching the market soon. Nomifensine is currently available from Hoechst-Roussel under the name Alival outside the United States and will be available in this country under the name Merital.

Merital is chemically different from other antidepressant drugs and has some unique properties. Side effects are few and the drug is rarely fatal if an overdose is taken. This drug, like the others, prolongs the action of the neurotransmitters in the brain, but it takes a broader swath, including one additional chemical, dopamine. This may be the reason that nomifensine has beneficial effects against Parkinson's disease.

Other promising drugs still being tested are zimelidine, diclofensine, flumezapine, and ideloxine. Once again, they aren't any more effective, but they are much less toxic. Diclofensine seems to be the best, with virtually no effects on the heart and no sedative effect either. In fact, the major problem is the energizing effect experienced by people taking it.

While researchers look for antidepressant drugs that can also relieve anxiety, there is at least one antianxiety drug that seems to work against depression as well. That drug is alpazolam, a chemical relative of Valium.

One more drug that may ultimately find some use is amperozide, currently classified as a drug to be used against aggression. It also is turning out to be a potent pain killer and may see use for that purpose as well.

An interesting, although unaccepted approach to treating depression has been singlehandedly promoted by Wall Street businessman Jack Dreyfus. Dreyfus claims that phenytoin, sold as an anticonvulsant drug named Dilantin by the Parke-Davis Company, can effectively treat depression. Dreyfus himself claims to have been cured by the drug.

His idea is that by stabilizing nerves, much as it does in preventing epileptic seizures, Dilantin can also stabilize the abnormal goings on in the nerves that are the cause of the depression. Even though there is little hard evidence to support his claims, it is possible a small number of people could benefit from the drug. Other medical experts, however, think the idea is potentially dangerous.

Unfortunately, Dreyfus' expensive effort to promote and prove his theory about Dilantin (including a book published on this matter) has been largely ignored. A final answer on the usefulness of Dilantin for depression may be a long time in coming.

Insanity on Trial

The notion that mental illness, or insanity, is an involuntary medical problem is also the basis for allowing a defense of insanity in a court of law. The most talked about recent case involved would-be presidential assassin John Hinckley, Jr. The psychiatrists who testified at Hinckley's trial disagreed on the specific diagnosis of his problem, but there was general agreement that Hinckley had not received proper treatment. The consensus is that he suffered from a form of schizophrenia and was deeply depressed for months before the assassination attempt on Ronald Reagan.

What if Hinckley had been given proper treatment for his condition? The drugs covered in this chapter are capable of treating just such severe depression. They may well have been able to stabilize Hinckley's mental state. And what if he had received the drugs and had still tried to kill the President? Would the fact that he had received state-of-the-art therapy have made a difference to the jury? We will probably never learn the answers to those questions. Courts have tended to take therapy into consideration, but then again juries usually have rejected the insanity plea anyway.

Continuing advances in drugs to treat mental illness offer hope of preventing self-destructive and desperate criminal acts in some individuals. Drug therapy may be a good defense against insanity.

34

MOTION SICKNESS PREVENTION: STICK IT BEHIND YOUR EAR

Some people suffer it while riding in cars, some on trains, boats, or airplanes, and even briefly on an elevator or long escalator. It is motion sickness, and while it is hardly a life-threatening disorder, it can be rather annoying and discomforting to the many sufferers.

Drugs to treat it have been around for a long time, but now there is a novel method of motion sickness prevention you can use simply by placing a small Band-Aid-like patch behind your ear.

The product, Transderm-Scop (formerly Transderm-V), is a flexible disk made of layers of plastic, about an inch across, which sticks to the skin. You place the patch behind the ear and it will slowly release a drug which prevents motion sickness for up to three days.

The active ingredient is scopolamine, long known to be the single most effective agent to treat motion sickness when taken by a needle injection. Since few people are willing to go this far, the most effective motion sickness drug was not widely used until now. The unique aspect of this new product is not the drug itself but rather the patch-behind-the-ear approach.

Drug therapy in general has proven effective in preventing motion sickness, although drugs haven't done so well in treating the *symptoms* of motion sickness once they appear. Those symptoms usually include nausea and vomiting, in addition to a generally disoriented feeling. The repetitive movement of a car or boat causes the body to lose its normal sense of balance, which in turn leads to discomfort.

Antihistamines such as dimenhydrinate (Dramamine) and meclizine (Antivert and Bonine) have been the mainstays of drugs available for treating motion sickness. They are effective if taken orally thirty to sixty minutes before starting a trip but they sometimes do not last long. Doses of dimenhydrinate are needed every four hours and meclizine must be taken at least once a day. Antihistamines are notorious for producing drowsiness in most people, often an unacceptable side effect when traveling.

Scopolamine, the active drug that enters the body through the new disks, is not without side effects of its own. Many studies have proven it effective, but the drug can cause a dry mouth, blurred vision, and some drowsiness. These are easily tolerated by most patients and will reverse when the patch is removed.

The Transderm-Scop patch, which is about the thickness of a dime, is actually a four-layer plastic membrane that controls how fast the drug passes into your body. Over a period of three days it will release 0.5 milligrams of scopolamine, compared to a standard oral dose of about 0.1 milligrams.

Don't try to put the patch anywhere except behind the ear, however. This is the region of the body that controls the motion disorder, so by placing it behind the ear it goes directly to where it is most needed. Placed elsewhere, the drug would have to travel too far to be of much use.

Taking drugs through the skin, a method called transdermal, can be especially good for people who have trouble swallowing pills. Initially, the drug will be absorbed into the body more slowly than if taken orally, so the motion sickness disk should be applied two to four hours ahead of time.

Some precautions: While studies have shown scopolamine to be safe, it is also quite potent and not recommended for use by children or the elderly. Also, wash your hands after handling the disks and if you need it for more than three days, switch ears.

Because of these precautions Transderm-Scop is presently available only by prescription. And while effective, it is still not an ideal anti-nausea drug. Should research on another product called domperidone prove successful, however, such an ideal drug may soon be available. This drug is currently undergoing clinical trials and will be marketed by Janssen Pharmaceutica, a subsidiary of Johnson & Johnson. It seems to work specifically on the nausea site in the brain and lacks most of the adverse effects seen with other such drugs.

35

PAIN RELIEF:
A NEW ERA BEGINS

New Non-Narcotic Pain Killers

The medical profession, along with pain sufferers everywhere, has long sought a potent pain reliever that is not habit-forming . . . and with good reason. Pain is the most common reason people seek medical help, and treating pain continues to be a major focus of drug therapy, and of consumer spending on drugs.

The habit-forming pain killers—narcotics such as morphine, codeine, and meperidine (Demerol)—are terrific for relieving pain. But over the long term the human body develops a tolerance to the drug, which forces a patient to take increasingly higher doses to get the same amount of relief. Ultimately, this leads to addiction.

On the other hand, today's nonprescription, non-narcotic pain relievers such as aspirin and acetaminophen (also known as Tylenol or Anacin 3, and an ingredient in Excedrin), are not addictive. Neither are naproxen, ibuprofen, and fenoprofen, three non-narcotic prescription pain relievers, but they're all only good against mild to moderate pain. The ideal pain killer (known as an analgesic to your doctor or pharmacist) would combine the potency of the narcotics with the nonaddictive qualities of the others.

Until recently, everything new that came along turned out to be addictive. And although the strongest and most effective pain killers continue to be the narcotics, a twenty-year search for a better aspirin, something more effective and with fewer side effects on the stomach, has begun to pay off. Several new potent non-narcotic pain relievers have hit the market.

One such product is called diflunisal, sold under the trade name Dolobid. The FDA has classified it as a "non-narcotic, long-lasting pain killer." Several studies have shown it to be more effective against pain than aspirin or acetaminophen.

Although the government has given its seal of approval to the drug only for treating pain, diflunisal—like its chemical cousin aspirin—is also an anti-inflammatory agent. Further research and testing are expected to prove its usefulness in treating medical conditions that involve inflammation, such as rheumatoid arthritis.

In fact, the drug is geared largely towards replacing aspirin as one of the mainstays of drug therapy for millions of arthritis sufferers. The problem has been that most people with arthritis must take large and even massive doses of aspirin to feel any beneficial effect, and large doses of aspirin can be a potent stomach irritant.

The makers of Dolobid have apparently achieved their goal of producing an analgesic and anti-inflammatory agent which causes less stomach irritation than aspirin. And its effects last from eight to twelve hours. But the drug is not without other side effects and, as a result, is available only by prescription. Between three and nine percent of patients receiving this drug may experience some nausea, stomach pain, diarrhea, headaches, or other ill effects.

Research has shown that diflunisal relieves pain as well as the narcotic codeine, and is better than propoxyphene (Darvon), or aspirin. With its kinship to aspirin, diflunisal is not a narcotic and tolerance, habituation, and addiction are not problems.

The other attraction of this new drug is the length of time it continues to work. Pain sufferers need only take diflunisal twice a day to maintain a continuous level of relief. Aspirin, codeine, or

Darvon, on the other hand, must be taken four to six times daily to keep the same level of relief.

Just how diflunisal works isn't known for certain. Like aspirin, it inhibits the formation of certain chemicals, called prostaglandins, which are involved in producing pain and inflammation. As with all pain relievers, it is important to remember that these drugs do not treat the cause of the problem, just one of the symptoms— pain. The lessening of pain should not cause delay in the proper treatment for the root of the problem.

Another drug, zomepirac, sold under the trade name Zomax, (but recently taken off the market) is believed to be the first non-narcotic painkiller whose effectiveness approaches that of the narcotics codeine and morphine.

Zomepirac, too, was geared towards the lucrative arthritis trade. And preliminary research showed it to be more effective than many current agents in relieving the joint pain and other symptoms of this chronic disease. When compared to Dolobid, Zomax was found to take effect more quickly, but the effect did not last as long.

Although Zomax was promoted as having few side effects, it appears that as many as twelve percent of the people taking it experienced nausea which can progress into vomiting. There is also a possibility that the drug causes kidney damage in some people, and its other side effects may include dizziness and urinary tract infections.

In early 1983 there was a scare involving Zomax and potentially severe, and even deadly allergic reactions it might cause. The McNeil Pharmaceutical Co., a Johnson & Johnson subsidiary that makes the drug, was alarmed enough to temporarily withdraw Zomax from the market.

McNeil had documented some eleven hundred allergic reactions to Zomax by early 1983, including five fatal reactions. The company was already discussing changes in the label warning with the FDA when television reports of allergic reactions to Zomax surfaced. When you consider that over fifteen million prescriptions for Zomax were written, the incidence of severe allergic reactions comes out to be about 0.01 percent, twice the rate of related drugs, but one-fourth that of penicillin. The FDA initially didn't seem too concerned about the drug itself, but was afraid that doctors may have been overusing it. As Zomax's problems mounted, it was questionable whether it would return to the market.

It's still a highly effective non-narcotic pain killer, and will probably be used for many types of pain, including strains, sprains, fractures and dysmennorhea—a particularly painful menstrual cycle suffered by some women.

Although the precise clinical application and therapeutic niche these new pain-killing agents will occupy remains to be seen, the early evidence suggests that their development marks the beginning of a new era in the treatment of pain.

The "Super-Strength" Illusion and Other Myths

America's big advertising moguls on Madison Avenue have done a terrific job selling the public on "Extra-Strength" this, and "New Maximum-Strength" that, but beneath the slick advertising and sweeping claims, there's little "extra" about these products besides the price. Make the pill a little larger, and maybe throw in some caffeine, and suddenly the product is supposed to get rid of your headache faster.

It is all an illusion created by the manufacturers. There is little real evidence that any of the dozens of pain relievers on the market—Anacin, Bayer, Midol, Vanquish, Excedrin, Bufferin, Arthritis Pain Formula, Cope, Momentum, Maximum Strength Anacin,

Extra-Strength Bufferin, and so on—work any better than plain old aspirin. In fact, what all the slick advertising fails to tell you is that in most of these products, aspirin *is* the main ingredient. The commercials often try to disguise that fact with euphemisms and tricky wording. What do you suppose "the pain reliever doctors recommend most" really is? Aspirin, of course.

Consumers Union (CU), the hard-nosed and much respected consumer organization that publishes *Consumer Reports,* has compiled a lengthy report on a drugstore full of pain relievers, most of which have big advertising budgets. The question CU asked: Are any of them better than aspirin? CU's conclusion, in a word, was "no."

Nevertheless, the effects these ads have had on the minds of American consumers—the result of half a century of pain relief claims—is amazing. Consumers Union, for example, cites survey results that many Americans are not aware that products such as Bufferin and Anacin contain aspirin.

Anacin, made by the American Home Products Corporation, has gone through plenty of slogans, not to mention troubles with the government's Federal Trade Commission. What is it made of? Just aspirin and caffeine. A couple of plain (and much cheaper) aspirin tablets taken with a gulp of regular coffee would give you the same ingredients. Yet, Consumers Union says Anacin is one of the most ingenious of the products when it comes to implying that its active ingredient is something other than aspirin.

Bufferin is another one. It contains aspirin along with antacids that are supposed to make it work faster and be easier on your sensitive stomach. Consumers Union checked up on Bristol Myers, maker of Bufferin, about those claims. The evidence they found from other sources was that neither claim could hold water.

Many people may still remember the initial appearance of another player in this game, Excedrin, in the early 1960s. Main ingredients: aspirin, acetaminophen (also known as Tylenol), and caffeine. Another example: the new product Panadol, which is being promoted as a great new drug from Europe. It's simply acetaminophen sold under a European brand name.

Actually, Tylenol itself was a big success story—at least until the poisoned Tylenol capsules appeared in 1982. It had grabbed away a big chunk of the pain-killer market that once belonged to aspirin, and according to some accounts, became the biggest seller of all health and beauty products. CU's biggest complaint about Tylenol is that it is too expensive (generic acetaminophen is much cheaper). And advertisers often ignore a major difference between acetaminophen and aspirin when promoting its use as an aspirin replacement since it doesn't upset the stomach: acetaminophen, unlike aspirin, doesn't fight inflammation. Thus, while it might relieve some pain in an arthritis patient, it lacks the far more important anti-inflammatory effects.

Beginning about the time of the Great Depression, and continuing right up until today, there's been a never-ending stream of new pain products introduced. And there's no end in sight. Not when, as CU points out, Americans swallow over $1 billion worth of these little numbers each year.

Since there has been no new nonprescription analgesic since the switch of acetaminophen from prescription to over-the-counter status in 1960, manufacturers have been kept busy finding ways to convince the public that their newest product is also better. Recent years have seen a tremendous effort to exploit the common-but-mistaken belief that if a little is good, more must be better.

This effort is most evident with the rapidly proliferating extra- or maximum-strength pills. This nonstop trend has gone beyond being simply misleading (it has always been that), and has become downright dangerous. Just because a product is available without a prescription does not mean it is safe at any level. Until the mandate for child-proof caps, aspirin was the leading cause of poisonings in children. Acetaminophen can also cause deaths. Overdoses damage the liver, leading to a slow, painful death over days or weeks.

Fortunately, an antidote for acetaminophen is available if the overdosage is treated early enough. But with the advent of more and more extra-strength products, such overdoses may become more frequent. No longer will 75 to 100 pills be needed, but maybe only 50 or 25.

In the final analysis, it is foolish to take more of any drug than you really need. Taking the smaller tablets may seem less effective, but it gives you greater control over how much you actually take. Since all nonprescription pain relievers contain nothing but plain old aspirin or acetaminophen, buying the less expensive, normal-strength tablets will give you just as much pain relief, along with the added benefit of increased safety.

Other myths have been promoted by the makers of the so-called specialty pain killers—the ones that are supposed to be especially for back pain, muscle pain, menstrual pain, and so on. Here again, there seems to be a dearth of evidence that most can do anything better than aspirin alone.

Price is another issue. The low-cost generic aspirin available at your corner pharmacy can cost less than fifty cents per one hundred tablets, while the fancy, big-name products may sell for over five dollars per hundred. But while you probably do not need all the extra stuff they throw into some products, all aspirin is not alike. Differences in stability in particular may affect how much of the active aspirin you actually get if the bottle sits around your house for awhile. A good way to find the best and least expensive aspirin or acetaminophen product is to ask your pharmacist.

When pain becomes too severe to be controlled by nonprescription products, it is usually time to turn to the more potent prescription drugs. But are they always more potent? In the case of propoxyphene (Darvon), an older, and now suspect narcotic pain reliever, the answer is no.

When first introduced, Darvon was touted as a potent, non-addicting, narcotic-like analgesic. We now know, however, that it is more than "narcotic-like." It is a narcotic, and addiction is possible. What is more, most studies suggest that the lowest dose commonly given is useless, while the highest dose works only as well as one aspirin tablet.

Curiously, most preparations of propoxyphene on the market also contain aspirin or acetaminophen. While this addition may help cover up the drug's poor pain-relieving ability, it does nothing to alter the severe side effects such as depressed breathing, the potential for addiction, and the recent discovery that it may slow down the body's ability to metabolize other drugs.

At one time, propoxyphene was even a favorite of drug addicts since it came as a separate tablet inside capsules containing aspirin, phenacetin, and caffeine. This made it easy to get in a pure form that could be injected intravenously.

Today, the use of Darvon and other drugs containing propoxyphene has slowed greatly due to federal controls, and evidence that it simply is not effective.

And, finally, the American public can, at last, say goodbye to an old pain-killing drug called phenacetin. Years after it was first shown to produce severe kidney damage in some people, the FDA finally decided to ban it from over-the-counter and prescription drugs as of August 1983.

Phenacetin was once widely used, mainly in a combination with aspirin and caffeine. This product was called APC, taking its name from the first letter of the three ingredients. With the knowledge that it could cause kidney damage, sales of this product plummeted, and manufacturers gradually replaced the phenacetin with something consumers are more familiar with: acetaminophen.

On the surface, it might not seem like much of a change since once inside the body, phenacetin is converted to acetaminophen anyway, but it did do away with the problem of kidney damage.

Finding replacements for phenacetin is hardly a problem, and one wonders what took the FDA so long to act. A few of the products affected by this action include: Darvon Compound, PAC, A.S.A. Compound, Duradyne, and Sal-Fayne Capsules.

DMSO: Industrial-Strength Pain Relief?

Strange as it may sound, dimethyl sulfoxide (DMSO), the solvent that is a byproduct of paper manufacturing, actually seems to work as an analgesic. It is not so much that it directly relieves pain, but it does have some significant anti-inflammatory effects that remove a major source of pain. Over the last several years, this effect has gained DMSO a considerable underground following as a treatment for arthritis and other aches.

Why an underground following? Because the FDA has not approved DMSO as a pain reliever. That means the DMSO you can buy in your local store is not of medicinal quality and may contain toxic impurities.

The discovery that DMSO has anti-inflammatory activity came pretty much by accident. Because it is such an excellent solvent, it was originally used to dissolve various drugs. Then it was discovered that DMSO could help carry these drugs through the skin and into the bloodstream. Suddenly DMSO was helping pave the way toward topical administration of many drugs.

Then several animal studies suggested that high doses of DMSO could cause eye damage. This scared the FDA, and human tests with DMSO halted shortly after its anti-inflammatory activity was noticed. Further studies indicate the eye effects do not occur in humans, and some testing has resumed. Although the FDA remains unconvinced about DMSO, the agency has approved the use of the drug for a painful inflammatory disorder of the urinary tract called interstitial cystitis.

Since the patent on DMSO has expired, and it is so cheap to produce, it seems unlikely that any drug company will want to spend the millions of dollars necessary to get DMSO approved as a general anti-inflammatory agent. And although DMSO apparently works, it is not without problems. It is applied topically, and since it dissolves and transports so many chemicals so well, any environmental pollutants present on the skin could get into the bloodstream, a very dangerous possibility. There has also been a report linking DMSO to chromosome damage, and there is no doubt it causes an unpleasant taste and bad breath in those using it.

For the foreseeable future, DMSO users will have to continue risking these dangers, plus the impurities in the product they may be purchasing.

Advanced Narcotics: Top-of-the-Line Pain Relief

Drugs such as morphine and meperidine (Demerol) have long been the mainstays for treating the victims of severe types of pain in the United States. They are among a group of drugs known as the narcotic analgesics and, unfortunately, they have some pretty significant side effects that have severely limited their use and also led to drug abuse. Those side effects include physical dependence, or addiction, depressed breathing, and constipation.

Scientists now know much more about how these drugs work, and the result has been the development of new products which are just as effective against chronic and severe pain as morphine, but with far fewer side effects. What's more, these new advanced narcotics rarely result in addiction if overused or misused.

Probably the most interesting of the new pain killers under study is called THIP. This drug is showing the potential for becoming the first totally nonaddictive pain killer that is as effective as morphine.

THIP comes from a chemical found in a poisonous mushroom and seems to work by a totally different bodily mechanism than morphine. Even so, it is highly effective and can be taken orally. THIP has been undergoing testing in Europe and if the side effects prove tolerable it could be seen in pharmacies in the United States by the late 1980s.

It seems incredible, but two other chemicals, isolated from human brain tissue in 1975, actually have many of the same effects as morphine. These chemicals, called endorphins and enkephalins are relatives of proteins. There were early hopes that these chemicals were the final prize in the search for potent non-narcotic pain killers. Unfortunately, it now appears that animals, and presumably humans, can actually get addicted to them just like morphine. Nevertheless, a stable synthetic derivative of these brain chemicals, called metkephamid, has now been tested in humans and may one day be approved for general use.

Researchers are now focusing on the role of these chemicals in various mental diseases. One chemical, called beta-endorphin, has been found to elevate the mood of depressed patients. It also seems to aggravate the symptoms of schizophrenia, suggesting that the abnormal production of this morphine-like chemical in the brain may play a role in these disorders.

THE NARCOTIC BLOCKERS

Some of the new pain-killing products can be traced to the discovery of a class of drugs called narcotic antagonists. The narcotic antagonists have the ability to completely block all effects of a narcotic drug in the body. What is more, they have no other effect of their own. A drug called naloxone is the prototype of this variety of drug. It is available in the United States under the trade name Narcan and is now being used to treat, and actually reverse all of the effects that go along with accidental or intentional overdoses of narcotics. Naloxone can also block the effects of the morphine-like brain chemicals, and some people believe this drug may turn out to be a weapon against some mental diseases.

Naloxone is a "pure" antagonist, carrying no narcotic-like effects of its own. But there's another group of drugs called mixed agonists-antagonists (agonist being the opposite of antagonist). Medical experts first thought these drugs could combine the pain-relieving potency of morphine with much less potential for abuse. But the drugs, such as pentazocine (Talwin) did not live up to that billing. Large doses caused nervousness, mood changes, and even some physical dependence.

Now there is a second generation of antagonist-analgesics that is being marketed in the United States. These second-generation drugs show great improvement in their pain-killing potency, side-effects, and lower addiction potential.

Two of these drugs are already available: nalbuphine, carrying the trade name Nubain, and butorphanol, known also as Stadol. Two others, buprenorphine (Temgesic) and propiram (Dirame) are headed for approval. They are available only by injection, although an oral form of Nubain is also being developed.

Even the conservative-minded FDA has left these new drugs free of stiff narcotic controls, and that should say something encouraging about their safety.

The phenomenon known as tolerance may also be licked by these second-generation products. That alone would be a major advancement. As it is now, patients receiving morphine must be given gradually increasing doses in order to keep up the same level of pain relief. That's because the body builds up a tolerance to the morphine. But cancer patients using Nubain and Stadol for as long as nine months have not needed a dosage increase. These drugs also have much less of an effect on breathing, making them far safer than morphine.

With attention focusing on these new products, a far older narcotic has also generated some headlines—heroin. A report filtering out of Britain claimed that heroin is a stronger pain killer than morphine, works faster, and has fewer side effects. Too bad those claims are probably wrong. Chemically, heroin is merely a more potent derivative of morphine. *But simple potency has nothing to do with how effective a drug is in achieving its therapeutic goals.* A higher dosage of morphine can relieve pain just as well as heroin, and there does not seem to be much of a rationale for legalizing heroin for this type of use.

Doctors and even patients are most often reluctant to use enough of a narcotic, for fear of causing addiction. Such fears should take a back seat for terminally ill patients, while for others the new nonaddictive drugs may be the answer.

36

PARKINSON'S DISEASE: BRAIN TRANSPLANTS AND OTHER ADVANCES

Once considered unthinkable, a transplant involving the human brain has now been performed by surgeons in Sweden. It was not, it should be quickly pointed out, the cinematic kind of transplant of an entire human brain from one body to another. Rather, it was a carefully conducted graft of tissue from the adrenal gland into the brain of a person suffering from Parkinson's disease.

Doctors were betting that the transplanted tissue would produce dopamine, a chemical that is lacking in the brain of a Parkinson's disease victim, and thus relieve that individual's symptoms of the disease.

The future chances for success of this radical procedure are unknown, but there is evidence that rejection, the bane of organ transplants, may not even be a problem in the brain. Years of research will be needed to find out more information.

The attempt at a brain transplant may have simply been the next logical step in the frustrating search for a Parkinson's disease cure. James Parkinson first described the disease in 1817, and its cause remains a mystery to this day.

Doctors do know that it usually strikes people in their fifties and sixties, and progresses slowly. A victim's mental abilities aren't affected, but the disease will cause the person to experience involuntary tremors, weakness, and rigidity that are due to the breakdown of an area of the brain that produces the chemical dopamine. Normally, the brain will release the dopamine when stimulated. The chemical then aids in smooth, voluntary movements. Without the dopamine, a person's muscle control is partially lost, and Parkinson's disease develops.

Other Steps in Treating Parkinson's Disease

Further steps in treating Parkinson's disease are expected, but unfortunately the advances being made still don't cure the disease. They merely relieve some of the symptoms.

Once doctors realized the lack of dopamine was crucial, therapy could advance. Since dopamine given orally can't find its way to the patient's brain where it is needed, levodopa was used. That drug will get to the brain and once there it is rapidly changed into dopamine. But as more brain nerves die, levodopa becomes less and less effective. The drug starts to wear off and symptoms return before it is time for the next dosage. Patients can also encounter an on-off effect where symptoms of the disease abruptly start and stop unpredictably.

Because of severe side effects, simply taking more of the drug is ruled out. Patients are given high doses to begin with because most of the drug is converted to dopamine in the blood before it has a chance to get into the brain. This results in nausea, low blood pressure, and confusion.

The discovery of another drug, carbidopa, is providing some help. When combined with levodopa, carbidopa allows its conversion to dopamine in the brain, but not in the blood, thus permitting much lower doses.

Another approach is to use drugs that stimulate the dopamine nerves directly in the brain. These are called dopamine agonists. The first drug of this type for use against Parkinson's disease was recently approved by the FDA. The drug, bromcriptine, had actually been on the market for many years but for an entirely different use in preventing milk let-down after delivery in women not intending to nurse.

Bromcriptine, sold under the trade name Parlodel, is by no means an ideal drug. It works in only half of the people who take it, and its main use seems to be for patients in the late stages of the disease who no longer respond to other drugs.

A similar drug called pergolide is showing great promise toward becoming the next drug of this class to win FDA approval. Pergolide is very potent and works for a long time. Patients would only have to take it once a day. In tests with severely disabled patients the drug reduced the on-off effect, and it may possibly work even better in less affected patients.

The old side effect bugaboo still gets in the way. In spite of that, however, a symposium on Parkinson's disease has rated pergolide the most promising new drug to treat that disease.

From new conventional drugs to exotic brain transplants, the battle against Parkinson's disease continues. As long as the battle continues, there's hope the disease will be licked.

37

PROSTAGLANDINS: BOOM, THEN BUST?

At the time of their discovery during the Great Depression, prostaglandins seemed little more than a curious new group of chemicals that were responsible for some biological effects in the human body. The prostaglandin family got its name because scientists first thought the chemicals came exclusively from the male prostate gland. They were quite wrong. Everybody has prostaglandins.

By the early 1960s, prostaglandins had been purified by scientists, and the idle curiosity exploded into great enthusiasm. Researchers discovered that prostaglandins seemed to be everywhere in the body, and were responsible for triggering all kinds of bodily effects at astonishingly low concentrations. The drug companies were quick to pick up on the potent effects of prostaglandins as well as the seemingly awesome potential for new drug products associated with them. Many firms plunged into research on these promising chemicals, although none matched the resources that The Upjohn Company poured into the effort.

Over two decades and millions of dollars later, the initial luster of the prostaglandins has faded badly. Only three prostaglandin drugs have been approved, and only a few others are still being actively pursued. So far, prostaglandins as successful commercial drugs have failed miserably, although with research continuing, there is a chance they may rise again.

From a drug manufacturer's standpoint, prostaglandins are tough chemicals to work with. The many different types have numerous and sometimes opposite effects in the body. A single prostaglandin may have several different effects and it is difficult to make derivatives that will only have the intended specific action. The unwanted effects on one part of the body may outweigh the benefits in another part.

What is more, prostaglandins are rapidly destroyed in the bloodstream, making oral drugs of this substance mostly useless. Since efforts at chemical modifications have failed to overcome these problems, and the expensive process of producing prostaglandins has not shown much improvement, money for this area is beginning to dry up.

The most useful of the prostaglandin drugs to make it is Prostin VR, an Upjohn product that received government approval in 1981. Each of the prostaglandins carries both a letter and a numerical label, and this one is known as prostaglandin E_1. It is used to treat blue babies—newborns with a rare heart defect that blocks the normal flow of blood from the heart to the lungs. Left untreated, blue babies will die within days or even hours. The operation needed to correct this defect has in the past been successful in saving the child's life only about thirty percent of the time. The problem is that the newborns are very weak and there's no time to wait for them to get stronger before performing the operation. With Prostin VR, doctors can now buy time for the baby, allowing it to grow stronger with improved blood flow to the lungs. But it is not a cure, and the operation is still needed, although the odds are now greatly improved, and about sixty-five percent of the babies are expected to survive.

The two other prostaglandin drugs, dinoprost tromethamine (Prostin F_2 Alpha) and dinoprostone (Prostin E_2) are used to induce abortions or to start labor in women who are past their due date. These prostaglandin drugs are effective in those jobs, but are not widely used.

Some research efforts to come up with a prostaglandin drug to treat asthma are continuing. One of the problems is that prostaglandin preparations are very irritating when given by inhalation, and researchers have not yet found a way over that hurdle. Since one type of prostaglandin was also found to block the secretion of stomach acid, it was targeted as a possible treatment for ulcers. But it causes diarrhea—a side effect that has curtailed efforts in that direction.

Other Roles for Prostaglandins

Among other things, prostaglandins are responsible for making you sensitive to pain; they are crucial for blood clotting; and they affect blood pressure. Since the prostaglandins sensitize your body to pain, it stands to reason that a drug that slows down the production of this chemical in the body would help relieve the pain.

That, in fact, is precisely what aspirin does, although it took scientists until the early 1970s to figure it out. It is also the way many other pain-killing and antiarthritis products, known as nonsteroidal anti-inflammatory drugs, work. Some of those prostaglandin-inhibiting drugs include: ibuprofen (Motrin, Rufen); sulindac (Clinoril); meclofenamate sodium (Meclomen); naproxen (Naprosyn); diflunisal (Dolobid); and zomepirac (Zomax). Several of these have also been approved by the FDA for use in women experiencing severe menstrual cramps.

What the future holds for the prostaglandins is still uncertain. The key observation that they are very active in the body stands intact. Research on the chemicals is continuing in some fashion at universities, and the 1982 Nobel Prize for medicine went to three prostaglandin researchers. Some type of breakthrough may be needed to revitalize this once promising area for new drugs.

38

PSORIASIS: MENDING THE HEARTBREAK

Psoriasis is a rather common skin disease that affects several million Americans. Usually the symptoms do not go beyond the visible red patches with silvery-white scales, although there may be some itching when the problem occurs in folds of the skin.

The FDA has finally approved a controversial, although effective, combination method of treating psoriasis. The treatment, going by the name PUVA, involves using a drug in combination with exposure of the skin to a certain type of ultraviolet light.

The drug is called methoxsalen, known also by the trade name Oxsoralen. It has been around for years to treat another skin disease, vitiligo, which causes white patches on the skin. The drug is part of a class called psoralens, which have the unique property of being able to make your skin particularly sensitive to ultraviolet light. Psoralens occur naturally in several vegetables, including carrots.

In the controversial treatment, the patient is given the drug methoxsalen, which is taken orally in a capsule form. The area of the skin affected by psoriasis is then exposed to the ultraviolet light. Anywhere from ten to thirty or more treatments may be needed. The result is a slowing of the abnormal rate of skin growth that seems to produce the disease.

The name for the treatment, as approved by the FDA, stands for psoralen, plus ultraviolet light-A: PUVA. Since the drug was on the market for a long time as a treatment for another skin disease, it was theoretically possible for doctors to use it as a treatment for psoriasis. But the lack of government approval made many dermatologists reluctant to do so out of a fear of malpractice law suits, should something go wrong.

Broader availability of the treatment could help, since psoriasis can occasionally become suddenly worse, entering what is called an eruptive phase. There is even a possibility of severe, life-threatening forms of the disease.

There are still many unknowns in this area. The exact cause of psoriasis is not known, nor do scientists understand completely why the PUVA treatment works. People can be predisposed to psoriasis through heredity, and millions of Americans suffer from the skin disease.

The advertising slogan "the heartbreak of psoriasis" came about because the disease is cosmetically unappealing, and the variety of treatments that have been used in the past against psoriasis have largely been failures for many people. Apparently recognizing that how you look can be just as important as how you feel, the FDA got around to okaying the PUVA treatment.

But the green light from the FDA still does not eliminate the highly questionable safety of PUVA. It is not the effectiveness of this treatment that has made it controversial. It is undeniable that it works, at least initially. It is the safety question that has raised eyebrows. Those who were helped at first seem to frequently experience a relapse of the disease, which means they may be taking the risks of accepting the treatment without receiving the benefits of a permanent cure.

The chief concern is the possibility that the ultraviolet light treatment may cause skin cancer. People who received the PUVA

250 · PILLS AND POTIONS

treatment have been found to develop up to three times as many cases of skin cancer as would otherwise be expected within a four-year period of the treatment. Premature aging, a breakdown of the skin, or eye problems are other side-effects that can go along with the treatment.

All that aside, dermatologists have predicted that thousands of psoriasis sufferers will receive the PUVA treatment now that it has received FDA approval. But because of the potential for dangerous side-effects, it should only be used in the most severe cases of psoriasis, and not for every skin outbreak that occurs.

Since current treatments for severe cases of psoriasis are also quite toxic and dangerous, the potential dangers of PUVA really don't change the picture all that much. One of the main products used for severe psoriasis is an anticancer drug, methotrexate. When taken orally, this drug slows down the rate at which your skin cells divide, which is the same intended effect on cancerous cells. Methotrexate has many side effects, and using it regularly for treating psoriasis could be very dangerous.

If the psoriasis can be controlled with milder treatments, drastic measures such as PUVA or methotrexate should definitely be avoided. Sometimes merely getting a little sun on your skin, or using mild lotions can be enough. The FDA's approval of PUVA recognized that this does not always work, however, and makes another effective, although hazardous treatment available.

39

SLEEPING PILLS: TOWARD A MORE NATURAL (YAWN) SLEEP AID

Drugs to Help You Sleep

With millions of insomniacs making up a lucrative market, pharmaceutical companies have done their best to assure that there is no shortage of sleeping pills in the United States. It is unfortunate, however, that all of the pills which do exist are far from perfect, and can have some very dismal side effects.

This is undoubtedly a key reason that doctors have drastically reduced the number of sleeping pills they prescribe for their patients. Today's prescriptions for sleeping pills have dipped profoundly from the high levels of the mid-1970s.

The best of the lot now available are the Valium relatives called the benzodiazepines. They, too, have had their problems, but two of the more recent products on the market, Dalmane (flurazepam) and Restoril (temazepam) are very quick, and relatively safe at inducing sleep. The advantage of Restoril, the newer product, is that it leaves you with less of a morning-hangover feeling, so common with many of the barbiturate-based sleeping pills, and also a problem with Dalmane. It lacks the hangover effects because the body is able to metabolize the drug more rapidly. In fact, half of a dose of temazepam is gone within ten hours while half of a dose of Dalmane may still be around after three days.

Another benzodiazepine sleeping aid expected to reach the United States market is estazolam, also sold in Peru as Somnatrol. It is handled by TAP, which is a joint venture of Abbott Laboratories and Takeda Pharmaceuticals, a large Japanese drug firm.

Estazolam is also rapidly eliminated from the body, with no apparent carryover effects or rebound—that is, it does not appear to lead to increased sleeplessness on nights when the drug is not used.

The truth is, however, that none of these drugs really brings about a natural sleep. Over time, relying on this unnatural sleep inducement can be harmful, particularly to one's mental health.

Scientists are just beginning to make progress toward developing a safe and more natural sleep aid. One big step forward has been the discovery of a chemical in humans which produces safe, normal sleep in lab testing on animals.

This natural sleep-promoting substance is currently known as Factor S, and can apparently be found in all humans. However, it exists in incredibly minute amounts, making isolation of the substance difficult. Purification of 30 micrograms of the stuff (about the weight of a gnat or two) requires the processing of 4.5 tons of human urine—certainly not a fun job.

With that kind of trouble required to acquire the substance, it should be pretty potent, and it is. Chemically, Factor S is related to proteins. Whether its action can be translated into a commercially available sleep product is still conjecture at this point. Its activity in oral form, which would be necessary for a commercial sleep product, is not yet clear.

Some synthetic compounds similar to Factor S, and which mimic its effects, have undergone testing, however. They have proven effective, but there is a problem—an oral dose would have to be a million times higher than what is needed when the drug is applied directly to the brains of lab animals. It will no doubt be years before Factor S or a related product might be available for human use. But there is now at least the promise of a more natural and more effective sleep-inducing drug.

Today's OTC sleep aids also deserve a mention for the simple reason that they are so bad. The main ingredients in these items are aspirin and antihistamines. The latter are there as an attempt to take advantage of the sedative effect many people experience when taking antihistamines. Whether or not that actually helps people sleep is open to serious question.

Until about 1980, methapyrilene was a widely used antihistamine in OTC sleep aids. When that drug was linked to cancer, manufacturers switched to other ingredients. Two chemicals, doxylamine and/or pyrilamine, are now the most widely used ingredients, although the recent switch of another drug, diphenhydramine, from prescription to nonprescription status, and its inclusion in Sominex II may change that. All have similar effects.

Aspirin certainly has no sedative effect, but the rationale of the drug manufacturers who put it in sleep aids is that pain may be keeping you awake, hence the pain reliever.

Natural sleep is extremely important to your physical and mental health. Insomnia may be frustrating, but using drugs to induce an unnatural sleep should only be a very last resort, and then only for a short time. If you have persistent insomnia, you should see a doctor.

Unrest Over a New Sleep Aid

A new sleeping pill that has been causing controversy in other countries has now been approved for use in the United States. The drug is triazolam, a sleeping pill that is sold elsewhere under the trade name Halcion by its manufacturer, The Upjohn Company.

Halcion is one of many sleep-inducing drugs referred to as hypnotics. It also belongs to the benzodiazepine class of drugs, along with Valium, Librium, Dalmane, and Restoril. Halcion, like Restoril, is said to eliminate the morning-hangover effect.

But Halcion, first marketed in 1977 and now available in some forty countries, encountered some vocal opposition. An uproar in England—fueled by a sensation-seeking press—came out of reports that Halcion can cause certain people to become severely depressed, suffer anxiety, hallucinations, and other psychiatric problems so acute that they are led to commit suicide. In early 1982, incidents in England broke things open. Both were suicides: one a seventy-seven-year-old woman and the other a seventy-year-old man. Both had been taking Halcion and both were hospitalized for taking too much of the drug shortly before they ended their own lives.

The man's son-in-law, a pharmacist, was convinced that Halcion had provoked the suicide. Stoking the fire was the discovery that the government of the Netherlands had pulled the drug off the market in early 1980 after allegations it contributed to twenty-two suicides in that country.

Based on case studies, a Dutch psychiatrist alleged there was a huge array of adverse effects from Halcion, including depersonalization, paranoid reactions, fear of going insane, depression and worsening of existing depression, aggression, hallucinations, impulsive actions, and suicidal tendencies.

Two of the commonly reported side effects—anxiety and depression—could be conditions for prescribing the drug in the first place, and not a result of taking triazolam (Halcion). Dutch authorities later said Upjohn could put Halcion back on the market if more explicit warnings were included in the drug's packaging. Upjohn declined and the issue went unresolved.

Halcion's backers say the drug's side effects are no different from those of the other benzodiazepines. Still, those effects are not to be taken lightly. The charge of "trial by media" was also leveled against Halcion's critics whose evidence was said to be completely unscientific. Of course, this would not be the first time the dangers of a drug were exposed by nonscientific methods.

The controversy hinged on the ever-present risk/benefit debate. When do the benefits of taking a drug outweigh the risks? Medical science has long known of the many potential side effects of benzodiazepines—angry outbursts, nightmares, hallucinations, depression. They have known of the syndrome "Librium Rage," where elderly persons taking Librium experience uncontrollable anger and rage. But compared to the far greater dangers that go with barbiturates, modern medicine has always considered the benzodiazepines safe drugs.

Corporations may claim undue harm because of the publicity surrounding such affairs. But a debate over the side effects and reactions is of benefit to the consuming public if it raises the awareness of the risks, whether or not the dangers warrant removal of a drug from the market. *Quite simply, taking drugs involves risk. There is always a tradeoff: results for risk.*

The controversy in England, where Halcion has been available for several years, centered, in part, on the dosage level. Articles appearing in medical journals say the frequency and severity of Halcion's side effects can be tied to the dose. The drug can also have a more profound effect in the elderly, which provided fuel for the debate in England over the suicides of the two elderly people.

British health officials, responding to calls for removal of the drug from the market, as in the Netherlands, argued that the approved dosage in the United Kingdom was lower than what it was in the Netherlands and thus was not a problem. But as one participant in the debate pointed out, drugs of this nature should be relatively safe at many times the therapeutic dose, given the unpredictability of an individual's response to the drug.

Study results reported in the *British Medical Journal* also showed a high degree of anxiety in subjects given triazolam (Halcion).

Researchers said the body's central nervous system makes adaptive changes when faced with the drug, as if to counteract the effects. When the drug is taken away, the induced changes in the patient's nervous system persist, resulting in insomnia and anxiety. It is known as a rebound effect, but what is happening is equally akin to addiction. The faster the drug is metabolized, the earlier the rebound, and Halcion is one of the fastest yet. At least fifty percent of the drug is absorbed in 8.4 minutes and peak concentrations are reached in a little over an hour.

The Upjohn Company, Halcion's maker, says the drug belongs to an advanced group of benzodiazepines called triazolobenzodiazepines that can produce sleep quickly without causing a morning-hangover effect. It does so, Upjohn says, because the structure of the triazolam molecule is different from other drugs in the benzodiazepine class (including Valium and Librium). The company's view is that the Halcion affair abroad is nothing more than "an epidemic of hysteria." Scores of countries that have approved that drug since the controversy broke seem to agree.

With an estimated ten million to fifteen million people in the United States suffering chronically from insomnia, the economic incentive for Upjohn to market the drug here was strong. Upjohn notes that one in ten Americans already receives a benzodiazepine prescription of some kind in the course of a year.

In the aftermath of sensational criticism of Halcion in the Netherlands and the United Kingdom, it has been said that the only thing really unique about the drug is the attention given it by the media. Still, there's nothing like a little media exposure to air all the dirty linen, as Eli Lilly and the FDA learned in the big flap over the arthritis drug Oraflex. (See Chapter 15, *The Arthritis Drug Wars*.)

Potential dangers, from whatever the source, should not be easily dismissed.

40

TOOTH DECAY: A VACCINE FOR HEALTHY TEETH

Cavities have now become a target of the pharmaceutical revolution, and the goal of eliminating tooth decay may be just around the corner.

Much of the credit goes to fluoride, an ingredient in drinking water and toothpaste (as well as some insecticides). But the real victor over cavities will be something new, something we have not seen before—an anticavity vaccine. That's right, a pill to prevent tooth decay.

The prospects for getting just such a vaccine on the market in the late 1980s seem rather good. Officials at the National Institute for Dental Research have reported on a vaccine that can stimulate the production of certain antibodies in the body that then go to work in stopping the buildup of bacteria on the teeth. Those nasty little bacteria, which secrete acid, are responsible for actually producing the cavities. Recent tests have shown that the vaccine can produce a ninety percent drop in cavities.

The Burroughs Wellcome Company, a North Carolina firm, is

257

currently working on this vaccine, although other drug companies are also involved in the race. If the FDA ultimately approves a product, each of us may start taking a pill once every six months or so to prevent cavities.

Tests on humans at the dental research institute found significantly fewer decay-causing bacteria in volunteers who took the anticavity vaccine capsule. Researchers stressed, however, that the vaccine would actually prevent cavities only in people who continued with other anticavity efforts such as brushing their teeth and avoiding excess sweets.

One possible alternative to the vaccine would involve the use of new technology to produce huge amounts of antibodies that would then be used in a mouthwash to prevent cavities.

In either case, fluoride will remain a good ally. The discovery that this substance, whose relatives are also used to treat goiter and rheumatism, could prevent cavities was more or less an accident. Children in Bauxite, Arkansas, suddenly started having more cavities when the town began using a new water supply that lacked the naturally high fluoride level in the old water supply. Further trials of fluoridated water were started in 1945, and the evidence is now indisputable that adding this substance to public drinking water is a safe, effective, and practical way of preventing tooth decay.

Fluoride's greatest benefits come if it is used *before* the permanent teeth come in, although children of just about any age will still benefit from fluoride treatment. For adults, it's another story. The usefulness of fluoride in preventing cavities seems to be far less certain, although some benefits may exist.

Toothpastes that contain fluoride also can be beneficial, particularly in areas where the water is not fluoridated. Just how this works is not entirely clear, but it appears that some of the fluoride sticks to the teeth to fight bacteria which cause cavities. Recently there have been improvements in the chemical structure of fluoride as it exists in toothpaste, and this seems to provide even better protection.

When used in drinking water, fluoride is deposited in the tooth enamel, thus making the teeth harder and more resistant to cavities. But too much fluoride can be harmful. The most obvious effect of too much fluoride (called fluorosis) while teeth are developing is the presence of small paper-white areas scattered over the surface of the teeth. This effect is called mottling and is caused by the abnormal production of enamel. Even higher overdoses of fluoride can produce black-stained pits in the teeth.

Since the levels of fluoride that can be harmful are only slightly higher than the levels needed to make teeth harder, the addition of fluoride to drinking water must be done carefully. The recommended level is about one milligram per liter, or one part per million (ppm). If natural fluoride levels are less than 0.7 ppm they should be supplemented, but harmful effects will begin to appear if fluoride levels get up to about 1.7 ppm. Even natural levels of fluoride will sometimes reach or exceed this level, and children drinking such water should also drink water from non-fluoridated sources.

There has also been concern raised recently over the level of fluoride in foods. It has become so common in food, particularly in the processing of baby foods, that some kids may be getting more fluoride than they need. If this concern turns out to be justified, some measures will have to be taken to decrease the public's intake of fluoride, after all these years of trying to increase it.

At very high levels, fluoride is even poisonous. Fortunately, even the amount of fluoride in an entire tube of fluoride-containing toothpaste (not all have it) is not dangerous.

41

TRANSPLANTS: REFUSING TO ACCEPT REJECTION

The amazing ability of our bodies to search out and destroy foreign and potentially harmful molecules is the main reason we survive in a world full of disease-causing organisms. At times, however, that same natural reaction to foreign matter in the body can work against people, particularly recipients of organ transplants.

It is this biological reaction that causes a body to attack a newly transplanted organ, resulting in what's commonly known as rejection. Safely halting rejection is still a major problem for doctors who perform transplants, and in fact it became so troublesome that many experts gave up on transplants.

But the recent introduction of a new experimental drug called cyclosporine (formerly cyclosporin A) is already dramatically shifting the odds in favor of transplant patients. With this new drug in hand, more transplants than ever are now being performed, and with increased chances of survival.

When scientists first recognized rejection for what it really is—an immune response and the primary reason for failures in organ transplants—they started looking for a way to stop it, or at least slow it down. Tissue-matching became standard practice. This involves a biochemical test to compare the tissues of the patient and the donor, with the idea being to match them as closely as possible. The idea is to fool the body into thinking the transplanted tissue is *kin* so it will not attack. A perfect match would actually come from an identical twin.

But matching has many limitations, so drugs are also used profusely. Several powerful immunosuppressant chemicals have been produced that can prevent rejection by blocking the body's defense systems. It works in reverse of the immunostimulants that fight off disease by beefing up the body's natural defenses.

But then another problem crops up. While helping to prevent rejection, the drugs also destroy the patient's ability to fight off infection. The result is that most deaths among transplant patients are caused by pneumonia or similar infections, and not rejection of the organ itself.

Cyclosporine, first plucked from soil samples taken in Norway and Wisconsin in the early 1970s, was intially pursued as a drug for other purposes. It turned out to be a failure. In 1976 it was put through routine screening and researchers discovered that it could suppress immune reactions in the human body. The key, however, is that it appears to block the specific reaction involved in tissue rejection while at the same time leaving the body's infection-fighting ability intact.

A Swiss company, Sandoz Inc., which also has a plant in New Jersey, makes cyclosporine, and calls it Sandimmune. It is an experimental drug, not generally available, but doctors can get approval to use it on a test basis. Quick approval is expected, however, as the FDA gave it a fast track route through the drug-approval bureaucracy.

One recent study at the University of Minnesota Hospital showed that patients receiving cyclosporine for kidney transplants had fifty percent fewer infections than did people receiving the older-type drugs. But rejection was still about the same for both groups— sixteen percent. With fewer infections, the people receiving cyclosporine could be released from the hospital sooner, thus cutting huge chunks from the massive hospital bills associated with organ transplants.

Other successful tests have used cyclosporine for heart, liver, pancreas, bone marrow, and even rare lung transplants that until now have met with little success due to rejection and infection.

Overall survival rates for liver transplant patients are now close to seventy percent, at least double what they were only a few years ago.

Like the other drugs used to ward off rejection, cyclosporine will have to be continued for the remainder of the patient's life, at an estimated annual cost of about four thousand dollars. That is not cheap, but it costs less than returning to the hospital all the time to treat infections, something that plagues patients taking other drugs.

So far, there has been remarkably little toxicity observed with tests of cyclosporine. Problems with the drug that have cropped up seem to be tolerable and can often be minimized by lowering the dose. Some adverse effects include liver and kidney damage, abnormal growth of gum tissue, hair growth on the face and arms, tremors, and depression. There have also been several reports of lymphoma, a type of cancer common in patients receiving other similar types of drugs that bottle up the body's defense system. But lymphoma seems to occur less often with cyclosporine.

For cyclosporine to work, the patient must be started on it before any rejection begins. Once the rejection process is underway, the drug is of little benefit. However, if the timing is right, it is an exceptionally effective and safe drug. Even though scientists are not quite sure just how cyclosporine does its job, its clear usefulness in helping organ transplant patients makes approval and further use seem likely. It is a drug that could alter medical thinking about transplants.

Ironically, now that transplants are becoming successful, there is a nationwide shortage of donated organs. It is not that people are not willing—surveys show up to seventy percent are—but rather that they never get around to signing donor cards or letting their families know they would like to donate their organs after death. The waiting list for kidney transplants numbers in the thousands, and hundreds more have died waiting for lung, heart, or liver transplants. Every state has passed the uniform anatomical gift act, which recognizes the validity of donor cards, so if you would like to help someone after you die, get this card, sign it, and carry it.

42

ULCERS: EFFECTIVE
NEW AGENTS

Despite the incredible frequency of ulcers in America today, the causes of this disorder remain a riddle to medical science. To be sure, the secretion of excess stomach acid as a contributing factor has been known for many years. But it is the only physiological cause with a definite link to this common malady. Why that extra acid is produced is not known.

Just how prevalent are ulcers in America today? It should be clear from the fact that the number-one-selling prescription drug (Tagament) is for the treatment of stomach ulcers. (That is: number one in dollar sales; it's number five in total new prescriptions written.)

Stress, heredity, diet, excess acid, and an individual's personality have all been blamed for ulcer development. But these things are difficult to alter and many play only minor roles in causing ulcers. Controversy still surrounds medical explanations of ulcers. In any case, an ulcer is a serious disorder and should not be self-medicated.

Antacids were once the primary weapon for ulcer sufferers, and as recently as the mid-1970s, an ulcer patient may have received little more than instructions to take acid neutralizing agents, eat frequent, small meals of bland food, and rest often. These orders still apply but there is much less emphasis on bland foods and far greater reliance on several new drugs. Surgery, once a frequently used alternative for ulcers, has dropped off drastically in recent years. The number of ulcer operations has been cut by more than half in the last decade. New and far better drugs are responsible.

The discovery, development, and marketing of cimetidine radically changed drug therapy for ulcers. This is the drug, first available in 1977 under the trade name Tagamet, that tops today's prescription drug sales. The reason: It has been proven effective in relieving symptoms, promoting healing of stomach ulcers, and even in preventing recurrences.

Cimetidine, or Tagamet, works by preventing the secretion of gastric acid. It does so by blocking a chemical in the body called histamine—the same chemical responsible for allergic reactions. In fact, cimetidine is technically an antihistamine, but it works differently and cannot be used to treat allergies, just as conventional antihistamines have no affect on gastric acid secretion.

Tagamet's major side effects include diarrhea, muscle pain, dizziness, rashes, impotence, and mild breast pain and enlargement. Tagamet may also inhibit the metabolism of other drugs. This raises the possibility of some dangerous drug interactions in the numerous people that take more than one medication at the same time. Some rare blood disorders have also been associated with this drug, but overall, it is quite safe. And although cimetidine was a giant step forward in treating stomach ulcers, the search for other drugs has continued with further success.

One of the other new ulcer drugs is sucralfate, which carries the trade name Carafate and is made by Marion Laboratories. It first hit the market in early 1982 and showed steady growth in sales from the beginning. Before it was approved for use in the United States, Carafate had been available in Japan for several years. The beneficial effects of Carafate, which is also a prescription drug, seem roughly equal to Tagamet's, and the cost is about the same. But it does work differently in the body.

In the stomach, where the acid is present, sucralfate will partially dissolve to form a thick, sticky substance which likes to bind to active ulcer sites. This substance is not an antacid, but is thought to work by forming a protective barrier over the ulcer, thus preventing further attacks by stomach enzymes or acid.

Unlike cimetidine, which on rare occasions has caused severe side effects, sucralfate has so far been free of harmful effects, probably because the body does not absorb it as it does cimetidine. Constipation has been sucralfate's only significant side effect. Remember, however, it is a new drug and has not met the test of time.

A single dose of sucralfate appears to last for about eight hours and patients need to remember *not* to take antacids, Tagamet, or food at the same time as the drug since stomach acid is needed to form the coating agent and food will interfere with its binding to the ulcer.

Even Newer Drugs for Ulcers

Tagamet has been so popular that it has become a household word in many American homes. It has been one of the most exciting drugs of recent years on its way to the top of the drug sales charts.

But Tagamet's Achilles' heel is its troubling side effects (noted earlier)—the bane of many a popular drug. Its reign as king of the drug mountain has been suffering an uprising.

One challenger is ranitidine, sold by the drug firm Glaxo Inc. under the trade name Zantac. Ranitidine seems to lack Tagamet's peculiar side effects, and while it may reveal some side effects of its own with further use, ranitidine has so far been shown to be a very safe drug. It could garner a sizable piece of Tagamet's drug sales pie.

Zantac (ranitidine) needs to be taken only twice a day by the ulcer sufferer, and that's another key advantage this drug has. Tagamet is usually prescribed for use four times daily. Some research studies have also given Zantac a slight edge over Tagamet in how quickly it heals an ulcer.

Zantac may avoid the problem of impotence in men taking the drug—a side effect linked to Tagamet—although the maker of Tagamet, SmithKline-Beckman, denies that a cause-and-effect link between Tagamet and impotence has been reliably established. But even SmithKline-Beckman is working on a new and improved relative of Tagamet. Called oxmetidine, this product can be given just once a day (going Zantac one better), and may not have the other side effects attributed to Tagamet. Other improved products under development: Upjohn has arbaprostil (Arbacet); Bristol has etintidine; and Merck has one called MK 208.

A far more surprising development came recently with the discovery that the newly marketed through-the-skin drug for motion sickness discussed earlier may be an effective antiulcer drug as well. A product called Transderm-Scop (formerly Transderm V), slowly releases an anti-motion sickness drug into the individual's bloodstream. In addition to preventing motion sickness, researchers found it inhibits stomach acid secretion as well, with dry mouth being the only reported side effect.

The drug involved is called scopolamine and was once used against ulcers. But it fell into disuse for that purpose because of its side effects, and the availability of a better class of drugs known as the H-2 blockers (Tagamet and Zantac are members of this class). Importantly, however, those side effects only occur when the drug is taken orally. When absorbed through the skin (transdermally) the drug does not seem to have the same side effects.

Tagamet's vaunted position as king of the antiulcer drugs may also be threatened by recent studies which show it can interfere with the metabolism of other drugs. Tagamet appears to greatly prolong their action in the body, leading to toxic effects. Such problems have already been noticed in people taking Valium, the anticonvulsant phenytoin (Dilantin), and, the antihypertensive propranolol (Inderal). There are also reports that commonly used antacids, such as milk of magnesia, Maalox, and Mylanta II greatly reduce the absorption of Tagamet.

A stranger side effect of Tagamet is the drug's ability to cause some men's breasts to enlarge. It is certainly not life-threatening, but definitely unappealing to plenty of male ulcer sufferers.

Elsewhere, the French firm Rhone-Poulene is investigating a new, yet unnamed ulcer drug that inhibits stomach acid secretion in animals. It is not of the same class of H-2 blocker antihistamines, nor does it work like scopolamine. Its unique approach could make it useful for patients who do not respond to the Tagamet-type drugs, although it is still several years from the market.

Recently, some new findings on how ulcers are formed have suggested new paths for drug research. Scientists at Harvard and Northeastern universities have found that dopamine (one of the chemicals involved in nerve transmission) and related drugs can slow the formation of ulcers and speed their healing. Somebody noticed that people with Parkinson's disease, who lack dopamine, have a lot of ulcers, while schizophrenics, who have too much dopamine, seem to be immune to ulcers. Putting two and two together, they concluded that dopamine can stop ulcers.

Studies on drugs such as bromcriptine and pergolide, already used for Parkinson's disease at high doses, have found they are two hundred times more potent than Tagamet. That means much lower and safer doses of these drugs may soon be the newest treatment for ulcers.

As modern medicine continues its attack on this problem of our high-pressure society, it may not be long before ulcers join the list of diseases considered "curable."

43

VIRAL INFECTIONS: STRUGGLING AGAINST THE BEGUILING VIRUS

If modern medicine has its weaknesses, fighting viruses is certainly one of them. Viruses are tough little customers. They are also killers with a maddening ability to elude capture and defeat by frequently changing disguises. Flu viruses, for example, make surprise attacks on the population every year.

The battle against viruses is becoming more frenzied all the time as scientists seek to bolster the meager stock of virus-fighting drugs. They are facing epidemic proportions of virus infections from herpes, to the flu (the informal term for the more serious-sounding influenza), to the common cold. (See Chapter 30, *Herpes: The Defiant Epidemic* for more details on drugs to fight that disease.)

The assault on viruses is showing headway, and consumers can expect to be armed with additional antiviral weapons soon.

Scientists, first of all, are now a lot smarter about what a virus really is and how it attacks your body. The virus is really a microscopic parasite that forces its way through the normally adequate defenses of your cells. Once inside the fort, the virus hijacks a cell's normal reproductive system, turning it to its own evil devices.

Killing the virus without killing the cell in which it lives after entering the body has proven, so far, to be too much of a challenge for the drug manufacturers. Incredibly, only about half a dozen drugs have been approved for use in the United States against viruses that attack virtually everyone in one form or another. Some are mild but some are life-threatening. And even these few drugs have very limited use.

Why do the medical people seem like such weaklings against a mere virus?

Part of the reason is the ability of some viruses (such as the flu viruses that establish a new beachhead every winter) to change so quickly. That explains why there is always some new influenza virus in the headlines, usually with exotic-sounding names indicating their foreign origins.

Even the new, highly touted drugs to treat genital herpes are at best only a way to ease the symptoms, far short of any kind of cure.

The makers of flu vaccines have to make a mad scramble every year trying to reformulate their vaccines to keep up with the changes in the viruses. The only thing more useless than yesterday's newspaper may be yesterday's flu vaccine.

Great Strides

This seeming impotence against viruses makes the latest developments even more exciting. Progress actually is being made on several fronts. Drugs that can *prevent* a virus from attacking, as well as treat an active virus, are now on the way. Longer lasting, more effective vaccines are in the works. And, new types of drugs that fight a virus by a massive buildup of your body's own natural defenses are now being used in many countries around the world and may finally be headed for these shores as well.

Keep your eyes open for one such drug in particular. It is called isoprinosine, or by several other names such as Delimmun, Viruxan, or Pranosina. It is a drug that can supposedly enhance the body's natural immune system by juicing up the natural killer cells against an invading virus. The technical name for this would be immunostimulant, and the branch of the drug field devoted to such things is called immuno-pharmacology.

Isoprinosine is available in nearly sixty countries, but not in the U.S. That aberration is subject to change at any time, however. The maker of the drug, Newport Pharmaceuticals International Inc., Newport Beach, California, has had a running battle with the FDA for many years over this drug. Although isoprinosine is recognized as a rather safe substance, the FDA has been unconvinced by the scant evidence submitted in this country that it really is effective against viral diseases as the manufacturer claims.

Elsewhere around the world, isoprinosine is used against all kinds of viral and nonviral diseases, including herpes, flu, measles, hepatitis, chicken pox, colds, pneumonia, and encephalitis, to name a few. Not very many prescription drugs, if any, can claim to be useful against such a wide selection of diseases.

Ironically, while the FDA was feuding with Newport Pharmaceuticals over isoprinosine, a prestigious group of French doctors and pharmacists was voting isoprinosine the greatest therapeutic innovation of 1982 in France, one of the countries where it is available.

According to Newport Pharmaceuticals, "A remarkable quality of the compound is the absence of side effects, although it has been administered to thousands of patients worldwide in controlled clinical trials as well as being in general medical use." Effectiveness of the drug is said to be particularly good in people whose natural immune systems are somehow deficient.

As more tests were being designed in hopes of getting the drug approved for use in the United States, the company was claiming that studies and actual experience with the drug in other countries have shown isoprinosine can cut back on recurrences of genital herpes outbreaks. It is still no cure, but offers hope of restricting the nasty herpes flareups.

Also of interest is isoprinosine's apparent usefulness against a rare children's disease, subacute sclerosing panencephalitis (SSPE). Also called measles of the brain, SSPE occurs when the measles virus invades the brain and it is most often fatal.

Proving isoprinosine's usefulness against this disease to the satisfaction of the FDA has been tough, especially since there are only about fifty cases each year in the United States. Assuming the drug works, the control patients—the ones who don't receive the drug in a controlled comparison test—would be condemned to death, raising serious moral issues.

If the clear evidence mounts, isoprinosine may be approved in the United States for use against viral diseases such as the flu and herpes. Doctors will then be free to use it for other diseases where there appear to be benefits.

Another New Virus Fighter

Ribavirin, another new experimental antivirus drug, and perhaps one of the most promising to emerge, also looks useful against many viruses. One thing it does not appear to be able to work its magic on, however, is the common cold.

Ribavirin's broad ability to attack viruses is hard to explain, but the drug seems to be able to block the virus' ability to reproduce. It is already available in dozens of other countries and is also being looked at as a possible weapon against herpes.

Toxicity tests have somewhat dampened the initial enthusiasm over ribavirin. It seems to slow the production of blood cells in the body and may harm an unborn child if taken by pregnant women. Some countries have been slow to approve the drug for general use because of the uncertainty over side effects.

Another variable affecting the drug's availability, but not involving the drug itself, is the financial resources of the company that discovered it. ICN Pharmaceuticals has been short on funds needed to conduct the expensive tests of the drug that are absolutely necessary before it could be approved by the FDA.

Studies conducted on American college campuses have boosted the claim that ribavirin is effective against the flu. The significance of those findings should not be overlooked. While flu vaccines exist, the need to constantly change them to keep up with the invading virus hoards is difficult. In contrast, a drug such as ribavirin seems to be equally effective against all flu strains.

A key to ribavirin's success, and a possible drawback in making it available to the public, is the way in which it must be administered. Although it's used as a tablet in some countries, its effectiveness in that form is vastly diminished. Inhaling the drug is best, perhaps because that is how the flu virus itself is transmitted.

Unfortunately, one of those simple little squeeze bottles is rather inadequate. Success with the drug has come by giving it to patients in a sustained spray of fine mist over many hours, using special breathing equipment. Few drugs are routinely used successfully by the inhalation route.

The Killer Kleenex and Other Virus Enemies

Other antiviral drugs—some old, some in the early stages of development—are showing promise.

Different types of cold viruses can number in the hundreds. And as we are all acutely aware, nothing yet on the market can stop them. The rows and rows of cold remedies on the drugstore shelf may do a little to relieve the stuffiness—the clogging of passages from excess mucus and dead cells that are victims of the battle with the virus—or other cold symptoms. But there is still nothing to prevent a cold attack or get rid of the virus quickly.

Since any effective cold fighter would be a financial bonanza, drug companies keep looking. One firm has been working on a way to plant a virus-stopping substance in facial tissue, hence the christening of the "killer kleenex."

A class of drugs called the pyrimidones is being worked on by The Upjohn Company, one of the big drug firms. Early tests have turned up good antiviral activity in lab animals.

Carbodine is another product showing strength against the flu, while arlidone, a Sterling-Winthrop product, has value against herpes and polio, which still strikes some nonvaccinated people every year. There is also a drug called phosphonoacetic acid which specifically attacks the herpes virus.

Since any drug capable of fighting viruses that cause the common cold must have an incredibly broad scope, some experts think the first mass-market cold-prevention drug will turn out to be an immunostimulant (one of the drugs that bolsters the body's own natural defenses against the virus). Isoprinosine, the Newport Pharmaceutical's drug, is mentioned as one possibility, should it become available in the United States.

Two closely related drugs, one that has been available in the United States since the mid 1960s and another widely used in Russia but not available here, have been shown in recent tests to be effective in preventing the flu. Amantadine (the American product) and rimantadine (closely related but less toxic) turned out to be effective in preventing and treating the main kind of flu that can strike in epidemics, influenza A. Additional tests are being run on rimantadine by Endo Pharmaceuticals. To date it appears that it may be the drug of choice to prevent influenza A. Rimantadine could be available here in 1984.

Vaccines, Still a Success Story

The dearth of drugs to knock out an active virus, and all of the scientific activity in this area sometimes overshadow the work vaccines have done against viruses. After all, the only thing vaccines have done is totally eliminate the smallpox virus from the face of the earth. No small feat.

This was, admittedly, an unusual virus since it could only survive in the human body. Through widespread vaccination programs, once the last human victim recovered, the virus had nowhere to go and simply ceased to exist. An encore would be difficult with other types of viruses, but proper vaccination schedules can now prevent polio, measles, mumps, and rubella. Reported cases of mumps, for example, declined from 150,000 per year in the 1960s to only 4,300 in 1981. Measles is nearing total elimination as well. A vaccine for chicken pox is currently being tested which may prevent shingles as well. Even hepatitis can now be prevented by a new vaccine (see Chapter 29, *Hepatitis B Vaccine Begins Its Work*).

Drugs that can get rid of an active virus seem to be on the way, all right, but vaccines to ward off some viruses in the first place are dictated by common sense. There still are no vaccines for some viral diseases, but they, too, are tempting targets for researchers.

Vaccines are available that work not only against viruses, but against some bacteria as well. For years, children have been protected against diphtheria, pertussis (whooping cough), and tetanus by a single shot called DPT. Although effective, there have been numerous toxic reactions, mainly from the pertussis. Recent research has produced an improved pertussis vaccine which should soon be available. Furthermore, the technology used for this vaccine may pave the way for numerous additional bacterial vaccines.

A bacterial vaccine, approved in 1977 but just now becoming appreciated, is effective against pneumonia. This often-forgotten disease remains the fifth leading infectious cause of death in the United States. Some of these deaths could be prevented by the proper use of this vaccine—a fact manufacturers noted when they advised consumers to ask their doctors about it in a nationwide advertising campaign.

Other bacterial vaccines being worked on include ones for Rocky Mountain spotted fever, gonorrhea, leprosy, and Hemophilus influenza or H. flu. The most promising results have been achieved against gonorrhea, and hope has been raised that a way may soon be available to prevent this epidemic disease.

44

VITAMINS E AND C: HIGH-POTENCY MYSTERY

What good is vitamin E? Its function in the body is not known, and there are no known symptoms of a lack of vitamin E. The closest that researchers have come is the appearance of abnormal blood cells in premature infants fed a vitamin E deficient formula back in the 1960s. Not much to go on.

There's a mystique surrounding this vitamin, including the widely held, although mistaken view that it can improve sexual performance in men. True, male rats lacking vitamin E become sterile, but a similar effect does not translate into humans. What's more, since the basic function of vitamin E isn't clear, the optimum amount your body needs each day is also not known. The federal government recommends thirty units daily, though others say it should be more like 200 to 400 units. But reports have surfaced indicating that in high doses vitamin E can be toxic, so large amounts should not be taken indiscriminately.

The latest theories have it that vitamin E acts as an antioxidant. That means that it protects fats in your body from chemical reactions that could damage them. In effect, it prevents them from going rancid.

Some studies have also shown that vitamin E can prevent toxic effects such as blindness in premature infants when they must be given high concentrations of oxygen in order to survive.

Since most of the foods we eat contain vitamin E, there doesn't seem to be much chance of observing the effects of a rank deficiency in humans. Its value in guarding against diseases remains in question. As an antioxidant, it is conceivable that it could prevent certain cancers produced by reactive chemicals. There's also evidence that vitamin E can improve the production of antibodies, increase blood circulation, relieve fibrocystic breast disease, benefit some people with sickle-cell anemia, and raise the level of a substance in the blood that seems to decrease the risk of heart attacks.

One intriguing idea is that vitamin E can prolong life. This is based on the free radical theory of aging. Free radicals are highly reactive, short-lived atoms or groups of atoms that have at least one free, or unpaired electron. It is thought that perhaps vitamin E can react with and remove the free radicals before they can destroy vital cell components, thus increasing the lifespan. Mice treated with vitamin E did indeed live longer *on the average,* but the maximum lifespan was not extended; there were merely more mice reaching it. This suggests that vitamin E's effect was not related to its action on free radicals.

Vitamin E remains a mystery, and consumers should be wary of new claims that are bound to surface. The main beneficiary of these claims may be the pocketbooks of those who sell the vitamin.

Vitamin C

In contrast to many other vitamins, some benefits of vitamin C (also known as ascorbic acid), such as prevention of scurvy, have been known for a long time.

Vitamin C is a water-soluble vitamin, which means that unlike vitamins A, D, K, and E, your body cannot store very much of it for extended use. You should take in some vitamin C every day, and the government's recommended dose is 60 milligrams. This is only an average requirement, however, and evidence suggests some people need more, particularly smokers. Many vitamin C disciples consume huge quantities of the substance each day, attempting to prevent colds or other disorders. Formal research studies have never verified the claim that vitamin C prevents colds, although there are plenty of individual testimonials of success in doing so. One recent study done in Australia found that vitamin C might cut the *duration* of a cold by a day or so, although it found no evidence the vitamin can prevent colds in the first place.

Fortunately for those taking vitamin C in huge doses, it is remarkably nontoxic. Still, there are some dangers. Since vitamin C is an acid, it will lower the pH of the urinary tract. Over the long term, this could promote the formation of kidney and bladder stones. People also taking sulfa drugs to combat bacterial infections will be more susceptible to a painful and dangerous condition called crystaluria where the drug actually crystalizes in the urine.

Vitamin C has been promoted as a weapon against cancer, even though there is no evidence yet to back that claim. But on the other hand, while there is no positive evidence for vitamin C against cancer, there is no negative evidence either and therefore, no reason it would hurt a cancer victim if other proven treatments were continued.

There may be more to vitamin C as a preventative measure against cancer. The reasoning is similar to that with vitamin E, since ascorbic acid is also an antioxidant. Vitamin C might work as a complement to vitamin E which is fat-soluble. This potential protective action remains only a theory.

Natural Versus Synthetic Controversy

A continuing controversy between health purists and scientists is the difference, if any, between natural and synthetic vitamins. Simply put, they are chemically identical. The body cannot tell any difference either. You are better off with whatever product you feel the most comfortable with.

A far greater concern has surfaced over the potency of the hundreds of different vitamin products on the shelf. A study done by one vitamin maker who was trying to check up on the competition found a vast difference between the strength claimed on the label and the actual amount contained inside the bottle. The potency problem applied to both natural and synthetic vitamins.

It is a well-known fact that vitamins lose potency on the shelf, and it is a good idea to always check the expiration date on the label of what you are buying. Apparently some manufacturers aren't being very careful about their products, so you might want to check with your doctor or pharmacist to get recommendations on the highest-quality products distributed in your area.

Sometimes lost in the vitamin craze is the realization that vitamins are potent chemicals. In a balanced nutritional program, they are invaluable. When used for other purposes, greater care must be taken to avoid poisonous effects. Vitamin A, for example, can be lethal in large amounts. There are documented cases of Arctic explorers who died after eating polar bear liver, which is extremely high in vitamin A. Vitamin A overdoses can cause sleeplessness, headaches, and can promote bone deformities.

New studies also show that lifestyles have a definite bearing on your need for certain vitamins: Cigarette smokers need more vitamin C; if you are a drinker, even a moderate one, you will need more A and B complex vitamins; if you have a high caffeine intake, that too may mean you need more B complex vitamins;

HOW TO READ A VITAMIN SUPPLEMENT LABEL

BRAND NAME
MULTIVITAMIN SUPPLEMENT
FOR ADULTS AND CHILDREN
FOUR OR MORE YEARS

DIRECTIONS: One (1) tablet daily as a dietary supplement.

ONE (1) TABLET SUPPLIES:	POTENCY	% U.S. RDA*
Vitamin A	5,000 IU	100
Vitamin D	400 IU	100
Vitamin E	30 IU	100
Vitamin C	60 mg.	100
Folic Acid	0.4 mg.	100
Thiamine (B1)	1.5 mg.	100
Riboflavin (B2)	1.7 mg.	100
Niacin	20 mg.	100
Vitamin B6	2 mg.	100
Vitamin B12	6 mcg.	100
Biotin	0.3 mg.	100
Pantothenic Acid	10 mg.	100

*Percentage of the U.S. Recommended Daily Allowance for Adults & Children four or more years of age.

INGREDIENTS: Ascorbic Acid, Vitamin E Acetate, Niacinamide, Calcium Pantothenate, Riboflavin, Pyridoxine Hydrochloride, Vitamin A Acetate, Thiamine Mononitrate, Folic Acid, Biotin, Cyanocobalamin, Ergocalciferol (D).

STORAGE: Keep tightly closed in a dry place. Do not expose to excessive heat.

KEEP OUT OF THE REACH OF CHILDREN

EXPIRATION DATE: NOV. '84

Manufacturer's or distributor's name, address and zip code

100 Tablets

This is the brand name of the product. Multivitamin supplements contain more than one vitamin and are to be used to supplement the diet. Terms such as "therapeutic", "high potency", "stress" and "geriatric" are generally associated with formulations containing more than 100% of the U.S. RDA for one or more of the ingredients.

Recommended dosage by the supplement manufacturer.

This indicates how much of the U.S. RDA, for each nutrient, is contained in each tablet, capsule or liquid measure.

The source or form of each vitamin in the supplement is listed in descending order by weight. In addition to listing the vitamins, this list may also contain ingredients used to formulate the tablet or capsule.

All supplements should be stored this way in their original containers.

The product should be used before this date.

The manufacturer or distributor is required to put their name, address and zip code on the label.

The U.S. Recommended Daily Allowance (U.S. RDA) is the most commonly used labeling guideline recommended by the Food and Drug Administration. The U.S. RDA's represent estimated amounts of nutrients needed every day by healthy people. By appearing on dietary supplement labels, they provide consumers with a means to compare the vitamin content of a product to the daily needs of adults and children four or more years of age. Minimum Daily Requirement (MDR) is a measurement that may sometimes appear on a supplement label. The MDR measurement, however, contains vitamin requirement levels that are out-of-date and do not include as many nutrients as the U.S. RDA.

International Unit is a form of measurement for fat-soluble vitamins — A, D, and E. Fat-soluble vitamins occur in different biological forms. "I.U." serves as one standard measurement which takes these variations into account.

Water-soluble vitamins — C and the B-complex — are measured in milligrams (mg.) and micrograms (mcg.). A milligram is equal to one thousandth of a gram; a microgram is one millionth of a gram. There are 28 grams in one ounce.

All dietary supplements should be kept out of the reach of children.

The manufacturer is required to indicate the quantity of tablets or capsules in the bottle.

and, of course, if you are on a diet you need special care in supplementing your vitamin intake.

Nutritionists are also sounding a warning that many Americans do not get enough zinc in their diet. This element is critical for fertility and sexual maturity (sperm has a high zinc concentration). You may need it to help fight infections, for production of proteins, and to speed wound healing. Seafood, eggs, poultry, meat, liver, and milk are all good sources.

INDEX

memory loss, 216–218
mental illness, 219–224
meperidine, 228, 237
Merital (nomifensine), 222
Metamucil, 23, 154
Metaprel (metaproterenol), 19, 120
metaproterenol (Alupent, Metaprel), 19, 21
methapyrilene, 253
methotrexate, 131
methoxsalen, 248
methyldopa, 11, 197
metoprolol, 182
mexiletine, 192
Mezlin (mezlocillin), 89
mezlocillin, 86, 89
miconazole, 21
Midamor (amiloride), 199
Midol, 231
Minipress (prazosin), 50, 196
minoxidil (Loniten), 59
Momentum, 231
minoxidil, 195
monobactams, 92
Monocid (cefonicid), 88
morphine, 228, 237
Motilium (domperidone), 132
motion sickness, 225–227
Motrin (ibuprofen), 6, 43, 49, 104, 246
moxalactam, 91
Moxam (moxalactam), 88
Mutamycin, 131
Mylanta II, 268

nabilone (Cesamet), 132
nadolol, 182, 185
nalbuphine, 239
Nalfon, 106
naloxone, 238
Naprosyn (naproxen), 50, 106, 228, 246
naproxen, 246

Narcan (naloxone), 238
netilmicin (Netromycin), 89, 90
nicardipine, 181
nifedipine, 178
nisoldipine, 195
nitrendipine, 195
Nitro-Dur, 181
Nitrodisc, 181
nitroglycerin, 178
Nizoral (ketoconazole), 170
nomifensine, 222
nonsteroidal anti-inflammatory drugs, 11
Normodyne (labetolol), 197
NSAIDs, 106
Nubain (nalbuphine), 239
NutraSweet, 167
nystatin, 21

O-demethyl fortimicin, 90
Ocusert, 31
Oncovin, 131
Oraflex (benoxaprofen), 39, 102–104
Oral antidiabetics, 11
orphan drugs, 61–65
Orudis, 106
Ovral, 50
Oxsoralen (methoxsalen), 248

PAC, 236
pain relief, 228–240; 'extra strength', 231
Parkinson's Disease, 241–243
Parlodel (bromcriptine), 243
patient medication instruction sheet (PMI), 7
Paxipam (halazepam), 97
penicillins, 12, 93; VK, 46; G, 186
pentazocine, 239
pergolide, 243
perhexiline, 181
Persantine, 45, 114